ESSENTIALS OF
Radiologic
Science
Workbook

SECOND EDITION

ESSENTIALS OF
Radiologic
Science
Workbook

SECOND EDITION

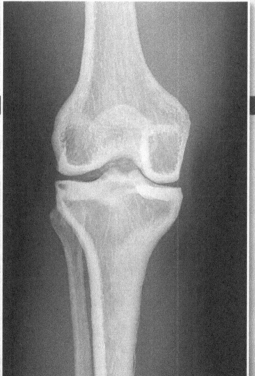

Starla L. Mason, M.S., R.T.(R)(QM)

Radiography Program Director
Laramie County Community College
Cheyenne, Wyoming

 Wolters Kluwer

Philadelphia • Baltimore • New York • London
Buenos Aires • Hong Kong • Sydney • Tokyo

Acquisitions Editor: Jay Campbell
Development Editor: Amy Millholen
Editorial Coordinator: Emily Buccieri
Marketing Manager: Shauna Kelley
Production Coordinator: Kim Cox
Design Coordinator: Elaine Kasmer
Manufacturing Coordinator: Margie Orzech
Prepress Vendor: SPi Global

2nd edition

9 8 7

Printed in the United States of America

ISBN: 978-1-4963-1729-2

Dedication

The second edition of this Workbook is dedicated to my husband, Tom, my children, Camden and Colin, and the ever faithful Kirby and Maxi. Finally, this workbook is dedicated to my parents, who laid the earliest foundations for the content of this workbook: To my dad, who patiently helped me with many hours of math homework—which definitely paid off! And to my mom, who named me because of her dreams to become a writer, but who instead went on to serve as an editor of my early writing assignments. Because of your time and support, this workbook is a fruit of your labors, too.

Starla L. Mason

Preface

Like the first edition, the second edition of the *Essentials of Radiologic Science Workbook* is designed to supplement the second edition of the *Essentials of Radiologic Science* textbook by Denise Orth. Each worksheet is correlated to a chapter in the textbook and contains Registry-style multiple choice questions, image labeling exercises of selected illustrations from the *Essentials of Radiologic Science*, and a crossword puzzle of important terms. Similar to the second edition of the textbook, the *Workbook's* questions have been greatly expanded, especially in the areas of digital imaging.

The worksheets can be used as a natural extension of the textbook for outside assignment purposes, and some of the labeling activities can be used to supplement and enhance class activities. Every effort has been made to make the material correlate to the textbook to allow for self-directed student learning, but also challenging enough for test review purposes. The crossword puzzles provide an enjoyable way for students to learn and/or review terms and concepts relevant to each chapter.

New for this edition of the *Workbook* are 20 laboratory experiments all geared for use in a digital imaging environment. Recognizing that film and automatic processing are quickly becoming obsolete and no longer supported in most energized labs—and that these topics will no longer be included on the American Registry of Radiologic Technologists' radiography certification examination—I have rewritten several of the labs for digital image evaluation and data collection. These include the labs on grids, field size, image receptors, digital imaging errors, and field size quality control. In addition, I have included brand new labs for SID and the Direct Square Law, Beam-Part-Image Receptor Alignment, Technique Chart Development, Digital Techniques and Dose Control, and Protective Apparel QC. All of the experiments are arranged in the order of the concepts as they are covered in the textbook and review basic physics principles in addition to some of the more traditional technique and exposure lab experiments. Each laboratory experiment includes objectives, instructions for completing the lab, tables or space for collecting data, and four to seven analysis questions to enhance students' critical thinking skills.

As Denise Orth states in the preface of the second edition of the *Essentials of Radiologic Science*, "...the difference between professional radiographers and 'button pushers' is that the former understand the science and technology of radiographic imaging. To produce quality images, a student must develop an understanding of the theories and concepts related to the various aspects of using radiation." The second edition of the *Workbook* has been developed with that goal in mind: the worksheets provide the opportunity for students to apply and reinforce radiologic concepts, and each experiment ensures that students remain active participants in the learning process while acquiring the critical thinking skills they need to be successful radiographers in an almost exclusive digital imaging environment.

Starla L. Mason

User's Guide

This User's Guide introduces you to the helpful features of *Essentials of Radiologic Science Workbook* that enable you to quickly master new concepts and put your new skills into practice.

Workbook features to increase understanding and enhance retention of the material include:

Registry-style multiple choice review questions

Basic Physics for Radiographic Science

1. The three fundamental units of measurement are:
   a. inches, feet, and yards
   b. mass, length, and time
   c. force, velocity, and weight
   d. length, width, and height

2. The two primary systems of measurement are:
   1. The British System
   2. The Grid System
   3. The Systems Internationale (SI)
   a. 1, 2
   b. 1, 3
   c. 2, 3
   d. 1, 2, 3

3. The quantity of matter in a body is the definition for:
   a. density
   b. pounds
   c. length
   d. mass

4. One object has twice as much mass as another object. The first object also has twice as much:
   a. inertia
   b. velocity
   c. depth
   d. volume

5. A large quartz sample has a mass of 500 kg on earth. What is the mass of the quartz sample if it is taken to the moon?
   a. 5 N
   b. 50 kg
   c. 500 kg
   d. 5,000 N

For Questions 6 to 10, match the unit on the left with the property it measures on the right.

6. _____ Joule   a. Time
7. _____ Kilogram   b. Force
8. _____ Meter   c. Energy
9. _____ Newton   d. Length
10. _____ Second   e. Mass

13

---

22   Part I: Physics for Radiologic Science

Image Labeling

1. Identify the subatomic particles and electron shells as indicated in the diagram below.

2. Complete the table of atomic mass and charge as indicated.

Particle	Mass in kg	Mass in amu	Charge
Proton	1.6726×10^{-27}	_____	_____
Neutron	1.6749×10^{-27}	_____	_____
Electron	9.109×10^{-31}	_____	_____

3. Label the components of the tungsten atom as indicated.

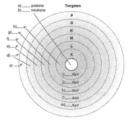

Image labeling exercises

Crossword puzzles

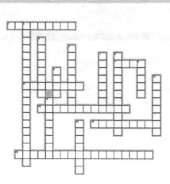

Crossword Puzzle

Across

1. Discovered natural sources of radioactivity
7. Most common material used as a radiation protection barrier
11. Discovered x-rays in 1895
13. Ability of phosphors to emit visible light when stimulated by energy
15. Developed by William Rollins to restrict field
____ boiling off electrons during the production of x-rays (two words)

Down

2. First digital imaging process introduced for use in static radiography (two words)
3. Material used for the filament in an x-ray tube
4. Required device to be worn by all radiographers to monitor radiation dose
5. One of the three cardinal principles of radiation protection
6. Device invented by Thomas Edison that allows real-time imaging
8. First documented fatality from x-ray exposure
9. Type of radiation emitted by naturally radioactive materials
10. Term for skin reddening as a result of radiation exposure
12. Material commonly used for filtering the x-ray beam
14. Roentgen was awarded the first Nobel Prize in this category in 1901

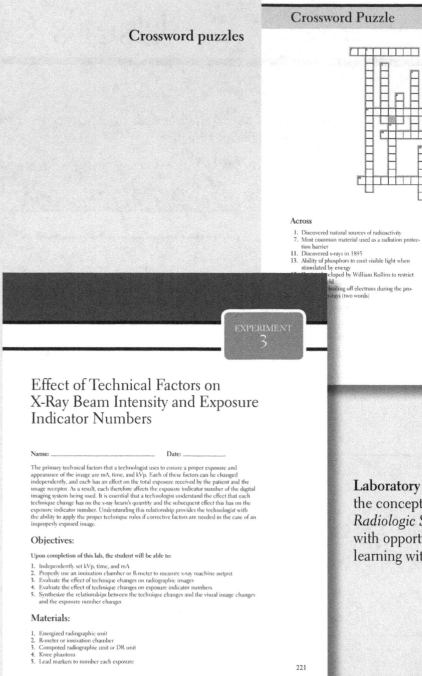

EXPERIMENT 3

Effect of Technical Factors on X-Ray Beam Intensity and Exposure Indicator Numbers

Name: _____   Date: _____

The primary technical factors that a technologist uses to ensure a proper exposure and appearance of the image are mA, time, and kVp. Each of these factors can be changed independently, and each has an effect on the total exposure received by the patient and the image receptor. As a result, each therefore affects the exposure indicator number of the digital imaging system being used. It is essential that a technologist understand the effect that each technique change has on the x-ray beam's quantity and the subsequent effect this has on the exposure indicator number. Understanding this relationship provides the technologist with the ability to apply the proper technique rules if corrective factors are needed in the case of an improperly exposed image.

Objectives:

Upon completion of this lab, the student will be able to:

1. Independently set kVp, time, and mA
2. Properly use an ionization chamber or R-meter to measure x-ray machine output
3. Evaluate the effect of technique changes on radiographic images
4. Evaluate the effect of technique changes on exposure indicator numbers
5. Synthesize the relationships between the technique changes and the visual image changes and the exposure number changes

Materials:

1. Energized radiographic unit
2. R-meter or ionization chamber
3. Computed radiographic unit or DR unit
4. Knee phantom
5. Lead markers to number each exposure

221

Laboratory Experiments relevant to the concepts covered in *Essentials of Radiologic Science* provide students with opportunities to directly apply their learning with hands-on activities.

Acknowledgments

I feel very privileged to be a radiographer and an educator and have been fortunate to witness the transformation of our field from its film-screen and automatic processing roots to a completely filmless environment. I am grateful for my first two radiography instructors, Quinn Carroll and Elizabeth Escobedo, who gave me the solid foundation in medical imaging I needed to not only be a successful radiographer but to go on and mentor and educate future radiographers as well.

I also want to thank Jay Campbell, Amy Millholen, and Emily Buccieri for the opportunity to work on the new edition of the *Essentials Workbook*—your support, guidance, and editing have been greatly appreciated.

Thanks also goes to the production staff who had the job of interpreting my directions and rearranging or redesigning some of the graphics from the textbook for use in the labeling exercises of the workbook.

Special thanks to my family, friends, and colleagues for their support and their encouragement to keep going. And I am eternally grateful to my biggest and best supporter of all, my husband, Tom. You unwaveringly supported me on this journey—and cheerfully helped pack my laptop while I worked on this project when we journeyed to actual destinations.

Starla L. Mason

Contents

PART IV: DIGITAL IMAGING AND PROCESSING

PART V: SPECIALIZED IMAGING TECHNIQUES

PART VI: RADIATION BIOLOGY AND PROTECTION

LABORATORY EXPERIMENTS

PART I

Physics for Radiologic Science

History of Radiologic Science

1. Roentgen's discovery of x-rays occurred in:

   a. New York, New York
   b. Wurzburg, Germany
   c. Vienna, Austria
   d. Paris, France

2. In 1896, _____ discovered that naturally occurring substances emitted radiation.

   a. Edison
   b. Becquerel
   c. Roentgen
   d. Madame Curie

3. The person credited with inventing the fluoroscope is:

   a. Roentgen
   b. Rollins
   c. Potter
   d. Edison

4. William Coolidge, an early radiology pioneer, made the following contribution to x-ray tubes and x-ray production:

   a. created a lead diaphragm for restricting the x-ray beam
   b. placed the grid in motion to absorb scatter radiation and improve image quality
   c. used a tungsten filament and hot-cathode tube and developed the rotating anode
   d. decreased radiation dose by placing a film between two fluorescing screens

5. X-rays are produced by an x-ray tube due to electrons being boiled off during a process known as:

   a. thermionic emission
   b. fluorescence
   c. radioactivity
   d. fluoroscopy

6. The best material to use as a barrier for radiation protection purposes is:

   a. aluminum
   b. barium platinocyanide
   c. lead
   d. tungsten

7. The types of radiation emitted by naturally radioactive sources are:

   a. alpha, beta, and gamma
   b. electrons, gamma, and x-rays
   c. x-rays, alpha, and beta
   d. electrons, fluorescent light, and x-rays

8. The first automatic film processor was developed in the:

   a. 1920s
   b. 1940s
   c. 1970s
   d. 1990s

9. Digital imaging and computed radiography were first used in medical imaging in which decade?

    a. 1950s
    b. 1960s
    c. 1980s
    d. 2000s

10. One advantage of digital imaging over conventional film/screen systems is the:

    a. ability to postprocess an image after exposure
    b. elimination of protective barriers in radiology departments
    c. reduced need for accurate technical factor selection
    d. ability to filter out scatter radiation

In Questions 11 through 20, match the physicist or inventor with his medical imaging contribution.

11. _____ Pupin

12. _____ Hounsfield

13. _____ Potter

14. _____ Becquerel

15. _____ Edison

16. _____ Damadian and Lauterbur

17. _____ Roentgen

18. _____ Coolidge

19. _____ Bucky

20. _____ Rollins

a. Invented the stationary grid

b. Discovered natural radioactivity

c. Developed first computed tomography (CT) imaging system

d. Used two screens in combination with film for dose reduction

e. Used filters and leaded diaphragms for radiation protection

f. Discovered x-rays using a Crookes tube

g. Invented the moving grid

h. Produced the first magnetic resonance (MR) image

i. Improved x-ray tubes by using a hot-cathode design

j. Invented the fluoroscope

21. Which of the following detrimental physical effects were noted or experienced by the scientists and physicians who first worked and experimented with x-rays and radiation?

    1. Erythema
    2. Weight loss
    3. Death

    a. 1,2
    b. 1,3
    c. 2,3
    d. 1,2,3

22. Which of the following devices helped to significantly reduce patient and worker radiation dose during fluoroscopic examinations?

    a. a lead diaphragm
    b. the use of a tungsten filament
    c. the image intensifier
    d. a Potter-Bucky grid

23. The three cardinal principles of radiation protection are:

    a. filters, screens, and grids
    b. time, distance, and shielding
    c. lead, aluminum, and tungsten
    d. aprons, gloves, and gonadal shields

24. When is it permissible for a radiographer or other worker to stand in the primary beam?

    a. when the patient is physically challenged and the image needed is critical for diagnosis
    b. when a patient is in a wheelchair and the image receptor must be aligned with the tube
    c. if a pediatric patient is unable to hold still or follow directions during an exposure
    d. never

25. Lead gonadal shielding is recommended for:

    a. all radiographers and radiologists when they are unable to stand behind a lead barrier
    b. all female patients
    c. all patients of childbearing age and younger
    d. all patients

Labeling

1. **Complete the table of Notable Dates in Medical Imaging by placing the appropriate year in the appropriate box.**

Date	Event
____	Roentgen discovers x-rays.
____	First application of x-rays in diagnosis and therapy are made.
____	Roentgen receives the first Nobel Prize in Physics.
1905	Einstein presents his theory of relativity and the famous equation $E = mc^2$.
____	Bohr theorizes his model of the atom, which includes a nucleus and orbital electrons.
____	Coolidge develops the hot-filament x-ray tube.
1920	Multiple inventors demonstrate the use of soluble iodine compounds as contrast media.
____	The Potter-Bucky grid is announced.
1922	Compton describes the properties of scattering x-rays.
1923	Eastman Kodak introduces cellulose acetate "safety" x-ray film.
1925	The First International Congress of Radiology is convened in London.
____	The roentgen (R) is defined as the unit of x-ray intensity.
1929	Forssman performs cardiac catheterization on himself!
1930	Multiple inventors present tomographic devices.
1932	DuPont adds blue tint to x-ray film.
1932	The U.S. Committee on X-ray and Radium Protection issues the first dose limits. Now the NCRP.
1942	An electronic photo-timing device is exhibited by Morgan.
1942	Pako introduces the first automatic film processor.
____	Coltman develops the first fluoroscopic image intensifier.

Date	Event
1953	The rad is adopted as the unit of absorbed dose.
1956	Xeroradiography is demonstrated.
1956	Eastman Kodak presents the first automatic roller transport film processor.
	DuPont develops the polyester base film.
1963	Kuhl and Edwards demonstrate single-photon emission computed tomography (SPECT).
____	Eastman Kodak presents the 90-second rapid film processor.
	Diagnostic ultrasonography enters routine use in medicine.
1972	DuPont develop single-emulsion film and one-screen mammography.
____	Hounsfield completes development of the first computed tomography (CT) imaging system.
____	The first magnetic resonance image is produced by Damadian and Lauterbur.
1974	Rare earth radiographic intensifying screen is first used.
1977	Mistretta demonstrates digital subtraction fluoroscopy.
1979	Allan Cormack and Godfrey Hounsfield win the Nobel Prize in Physiology or Medicine for CT.
1980	The first commercial superconducting MRI system is presented.
1981	The International System of Units (SI) is adopted by the International Commission on Radiation Units and Measurements (ICRU)
____	Picture archiving and communications system (PACS) becomes available for use.
1983	Eastman Kodak develops the first tabular grain film emulsion.
____	Fuji introduces laser-stimulable phosphors for CR.

Date	Event
1989	The SI is adopted by the NCRP and most scientific and medical societies.
1990	Toshiba presents the Helical CT.
1991	Elscint develops the two-slice CT.
____	Mammography Quality Standards Act (MQSA) is passed.
____	DR that uses thin-film transistors (TFTs) is developed.
1997	Swissray presents the charge-coupled device (CCD) digital radiography unit.
1998	General Electric introduces multislice CT.
1998	Amorphous silicon-cesium iodide image receptor is demonstrated for DR.

Date	Event
2000	General Electric produces the first direct digital mammographic imaging system.
____	The 16-slice helical CT unit is presented.
____	Positron emission tomography (PET) is available for routine clinical use.
2003	Paul Lauterbur and Sir Peter Mansfield receive the Nobel Prize for Physiology or Medicine for MRI.
____	64-slice helical CT is presented.
2005	Siemens presents the dual-source CT.
2009	NCRP Report No. 160, *Ionizing radiation exposure of the population of the United States: 2006* is published.

Crossword Puzzle

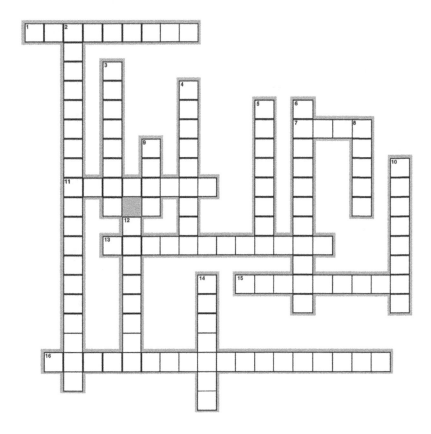

Across

1. Discovered natural sources of radioactivity
7. Most common material used as a radiation protection barrier
11. Discovered x-rays in 1895
13. Ability of phosphors to emit visible light when stimulated by energy
15. Device developed by William Rollins to restrict the x-ray field
16. Process for boiling off electrons during the production of x-rays (two words)

Down

2. First digital imaging process introduced for use in static radiography (two words)
3. Material used for the filament in an x-ray tube
4. Required device to be worn by all radiographers to monitor radiation dose
5. One of the three cardinal principles of radiation protection
6. Device invented by Thomas Edison that allows real-time imaging
8. First documented fatality from x-ray exposure
9. Type of radiation emitted by naturally radioactive materials
10. Term for skin reddening as a result of radiation exposure
12. Material commonly used for filtering the x-ray beam
14. Roentgen was awarded the first Nobel Prize in this category in 1901

Basic Mathematics

1. To convert a fraction into a decimal:

   a. divide the numerator by the denominator
   b. place a decimal point between the numerator and the denominator
   c. divide the denominator by the numerator
   d. multiply both sides by the denominator

2. Convert 2/5 to a decimal number:

   a. 10
   b. 2.5×10^0
   c. 2.5
   d. 0.4

3. To convert a decimal number to a percentage:

   a. move the decimal point two places to the left
   b. place the decimal point behind the first significant digit
   c. move the decimal point two places to the right
   d. divide the decimal number by 100%

4. If a structure on a radiograph is determined to be 1.13 times larger than its actual size, this can also be expressed as a magnification percentage of:

   a. 1.13%
   b. 11.3%
   c. 113%
   d. 0.113%

5. When performing a mathematical operation on two numbers with different decimal places, the number of decimal places that should be recorded in the solution is/should:

   a. match the number of places of the variable with the most decimal places
   b. always rounded to the nearest 100th (two decimal places)
   c. be a whole integer
   d. match the number of places of the variable with the least decimal places

6. Perform the indicated operation, rounding to the appropriate decimal place: 542.679 − 63.1 = _____.

   a. 479.579
   b. 479.58
   c. 479.6
   d. 480

7. The correct order of operation needed to solve an algebraic equation with various types of calculations is:

   a. addition and subtraction, multiply and divide, apply exponents, operations inside parentheses
   b. operations inside parentheses, apply exponents, multiply and divide, addition and subtraction
   c. apply exponents to each object in the parentheses, operations inside the parentheses, multiply and divide, addition and subtraction
   d. multiply and divide, operations inside parentheses, apply exponents, addition and subtraction

8. Solve the following: $(2 + 3)^2 - 7 \times 2$:

   a. 4
   b. 11
   c. 12
   d. −1

9. Evaluate the following equation, $4b - 2(a^2 + c)$, if $a = 3$, $b = 2$, and $c = -1$

   a. 53
   b. −3
   c. −8
   d. −30

10. The symbol and prefix for the power of 10 represented as 10^6 is:

    a. μ, micro-
    b. c, centi-
    c. M, mega-
    d. G, giga-

11. Milliamperage is one of the technical factors used when making a radiographic exposure. The prefix, milli-, is equal to:

    a. 10^3
    b. 10^6
    c. 10^{-6}
    d. 10^{-3}

12. Convert 250 ms to its correct value in seconds:

    a. 250,000 seconds
    b. 250×10^6 seconds
    c. 0.250 seconds
    d. 2.5 seconds

13. Calculate the total milliamperes-seconds (mAs) if the mA is 100 and the time is set at 500 ms to make the x-ray exposure:

    a. 50,000 mAs
    b. 50 mAs
    c. 2 mAs
    d. 0.05 mAs

14. 342.1 kilovolts (kV) equals _____ volts.

    a. 0.3421
    b. 3.421
    c. 342,100
    d. 342,100,000

15. To solve problems involving exponents, if a number with an exponent is inside a parenthesis which is being raised to another power, the first exponent value will be:

    a. added to the second exponent
    b. subtracted from the second exponent
    c. multiplied by the second exponent
    d. divided by the second exponent

16. Solve for the following: 3^{-4}

    a. 81
    b. 12
    c. 0.75
    d. 0.0123

17. Evaluate the following equation: $\dfrac{36 \times 10^5}{12 \times 10^{-3}}$

    a. 3×10^8
    b. 3×10^2
    c. 432×10^2
    d. 4.32×10^{-2}

18. Solve the equation: $\dfrac{(6 \times 10^3)(2 \times 10^8)}{3 \times 10^3}$

    a. 12×10^{27}
    b. 4×10^{24}
    c. 4×10^8
    d. 1.33×10^{-5}

19. To solve the equation, $6x = 24$, the first step would be to:

    a. find the common denominator
    b. add 6 to both sides of the equation
    c. multiply both sides of the equation times 6
    d. divide both sides of the equation by 6

20. If an algebraic equation is set up as follows: $x(2 + 5)$, "x" should be first:

    a. multiplied by both the 2 and the 5
    b. changed to 0
    c. added to both the 2 and the 5
    d. subtracted from both sides of the equation

21. Using the appropriate algebraic equation rules, solve for x in each equation:

    a. $4 = 36 - 2x$
    b. $2/7x = 14$
    c. $3x^2 - 10 = 45$
    d. $3(x + 16) = 152$

22. The advantage of using scientific notation in equations is that:

    a. once the values have been placed in proper scientific notation, only addition and subtraction is required to solve the equation
    b. it allows scientists to readily compare objects that are very large and microscopically small
    c. negative exponents are automatically negative numbers
    d. the speed of light (c) can easily be substituted into the inverse square law

23. If two variables have a directly proportional relationship, this means that if the first variable:

    a. increases, the second variable decreases
    b. increases, the second variable increases at the same rate
    c. increases, the second variable increases, but unpredictably
    d. increases, the second variable cancels out the effect

24. An example of an exponential relationship is the relationship that:

    a. kVp has with the density
    b. mAs has with density
    c. the numerator has with the denominator
    d. percentages and ratios share

25. It has been determined that a 15% increase in kVp is needed to improve the quality of a radiograph. If the original kVp setting was 65 kVp, the new kVp will be:

    a. 55 kVp
    b. 75 kVp
    c. 80 kVp
    d. 90 kVp

26. The formula used to determine the intensity of the x-ray beam when the distance from the x-ray tube changes is the:

    a. mAs calculation formula
    b. 15% rule
    c. mAs-distance compensation formula
    d. inverse square law

27. If the original distance from the x-ray tube is 36″ and the intensity is measured at 126 mR, what will the approximate new intensity be if the distance is increased to 50″?

    a. 243 mR
    b. 112 mR
    c. 90 mR
    d. 65 mR

Labeling

1. Complete the table for the more commonly used prefixes and symbols in the Powers of Ten metric system of measurement.

Multiple	Prefix	Symbol
10^{18}	exa-	E
10^{15}	peta-	P
10^{12}	_____	—
10^{9}	_____	—
10^{6}	_____	—
10^{3}	_____	—
10^{2}	hecto-	h
10	deka-	da
10^{-1}	deci-	d
10^{-2}	_____	—
10^{-3}	_____	—
10^{-6}	_____	—
10^{-9}	_____	—
10^{-12}	pico-	P
10^{-15}	femto-	f
10^{-18}	atto-	a

Basic Physics for Radiographic Science

1. The three fundamental units of measurement are:

   a. inches, feet, and yards
   b. mass, length, and time
   c. force, velocity, and weight
   d. length, width, and height

2. The two primary systems of measurement are:

   1. The British System
   2. The Grid System
   3. The Systems Internationale (SI)

   a. 1, 2
   b. 1, 3
   c. 2, 3
   d. 1, 2, 3

3. The quantity of matter in a body is the definition for:

   a. density
   b. pounds
   c. length
   d. mass

4. One object has twice as much mass as another object. The first object also has twice as much:

   a. inertia
   b. velocity
   c. depth
   d. volume

5. A large quartz sample has a mass of 500 kg on earth. What is the mass of the quartz sample if it is taken to the moon?

   a. 5 N
   b. 50 kg
   c. 500 kg
   d. 5,000 N

For Questions 6 to 10, match the unit on the left with the property it measures on the right.

6. _____ Joule   a. Time

7. _____ Kilogram   b. Force

8. _____ Meter   c. Energy

9. _____ Newton   d. Length

10. _____ Second   e. Mass

For Questions 11 to 15, match the quality on the left with its definition on the right.

11. _____ Acceleration   a. Ability to do work

12. _____ Energy   b. Change in distance over time

13. _____ Inertia   c. Rate of change of velocity over time

14. _____ Velocity   d. Applied to move or stop an object

15. _____ Force   e. Property of objects to resist changes in motion

16. A portable x-ray machine's mass increases (you keep hanging lead aprons on it), while a constant force is still being applied to the object (the cart), the acceleration:

a. decreases
b. increases
c. remains the same

17. What is the acceleration of a car that goes from rest to 120 km/h in 10 seconds?

a. 0 km/h/s
b. 8.3×10^{-2} km/h/s
c. 10 m/s/s
d. 12 km/h/s

18. Which of the following is NOT one of Newton's Laws of Motion?

a. the Law of Inertia
b. the Law of Action-Reaction
c. the Law of Energy Conservation
d. the Law of Force

19. To accelerate a 6-kg bowling ball at 2 m/s^2 requires a net force of _____.

a. 3 N
b. 8 N
c. 12 N
d. 24 N

20. During a dodgeball game, Player A launches the ball at Player B on the opposing team. If the action is the ball hitting Player B, what is the reaction?

a. Player B hitting Player A
b. Player B launching the ball back at Player A
c. Player B hitting the ball
d. Player B falling on the floor

21. A golf ball hits the green with a force of 49.5 N. The green exerts a reaction force on the golf ball of:

a. 49.5 N
b. less than 49.5 N
c. more than 49.5 N

22. A 5-N sack of flour is placed on a shelf 2 m high. How much work was done by the stock clerk?

a. 2.5 J
b. 5 J
c. 10 J
d. 2 J

23. Potential energy is the energy possessed by an object due to:

a. its momentum
b. its position
c. its acceleration
d. its shape

24. An object that has kinetic energy must be:

a. moving
b. falling
c. in an elevated position
d. warm

25. Which of the following is true?

a. a body with zero velocity cannot have any potential energy
b. a body with zero acceleration cannot have any potential energy
c. a body with zero velocity cannot have any kinetic energy
d. a body with zero potential energy cannot have any velocity

26. If velocity remains constant, this means that the acceleration of the object must be:

a. increasing
b. decreasing
c. 0 m/s^2
d. irrelevant

27. Calculate the kinetic energy of a wrecking crane if its mass is 1,200 kg and its velocity when it hits a house to be demolished is 5 m/s, the work done would have a value of approximately:

    a. 15,000 J
    b. 12,000 J
    c. 6,000 J
    d. 3,000 J

28. If the potential energy (PE) of a rubber band when it is stretched out to its fullest length is 0.8 J, what would its maximum kinetic energy (KE) be converted to (assuming a 100% energy conversion)?

    a. Less than 0.8 J
    b. 0.8 J
    c. more than 0.8 J
    d. none of these; there is no relation between PE and KE

29. Which of the following are examples of forms of energy?

    1. Electricity
    2. X-rays
    3. Heat

    a. 1, 2
    b. 1, 3
    c. 2, 3
    d. 1, 2, 3

30. According to the Law of Conservation of Energy:

    a. force = mass × acceleration
    b. energy cannot be created or destroyed, only changed into an equal amount of another form
    c. $v = d/t$
    d. all things with mass resist changes in motion

Labeling

1. Analyze the portable x-ray unit illustration shown. Identify each component of Newton's second law, by completing each blank with the appropriate letters: F, m, or a. Under each letter, spell out the full term and indicate the appropriate unit of measurement for each component: m/s², Newton, or kg.

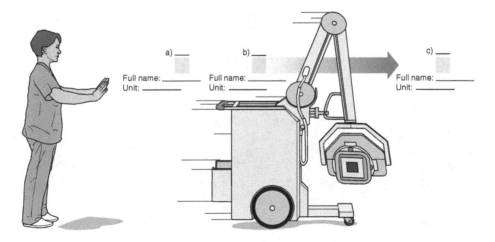

a) ___
Full name: ___
Unit: ___

b) ___
Full name: ___
Unit: ___

c) ___
Full name: ___
Unit: ___

2. Label Letter a as the "Action Force". According to Newton's third law, label Letter b as the "Reaction Force". Insert the value of the reaction force at Letter b if the action force is calculated to be 12,000 kN.

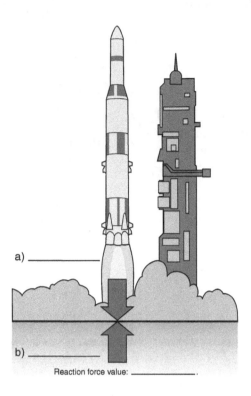

a) _____

b) _____

Reaction force value: _____ .

3. Label where the cyclist is exhibiting kinetic energy versus potential energy. In the last blank, complete the value of the kinetic energy if the total potential energy is known to be 1,000 J.

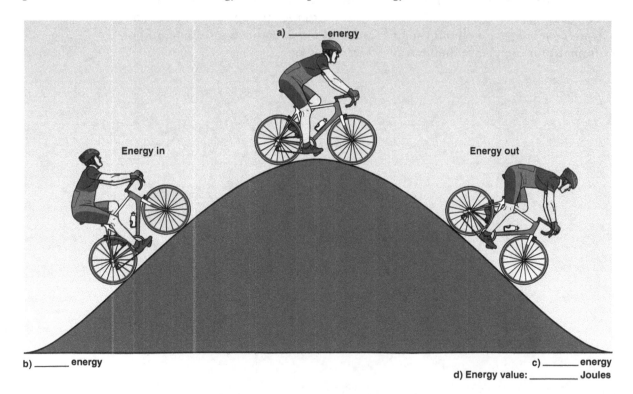

a) _____ energy

Energy in

Energy out

b) _____ energy

c) _____ energy

d) Energy value: _____ Joules

4. Label the types of original energy each object uses and the type(s) of energy each is converted to. For Letter d, label the type of energy represented.

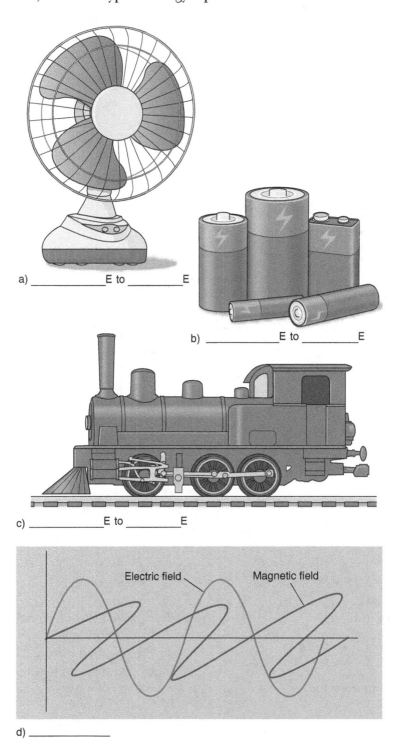

a) _____ E to _____ E

b) _____ E to _____ E

c) _____ E to _____ E

d) _____

Crossword Puzzle

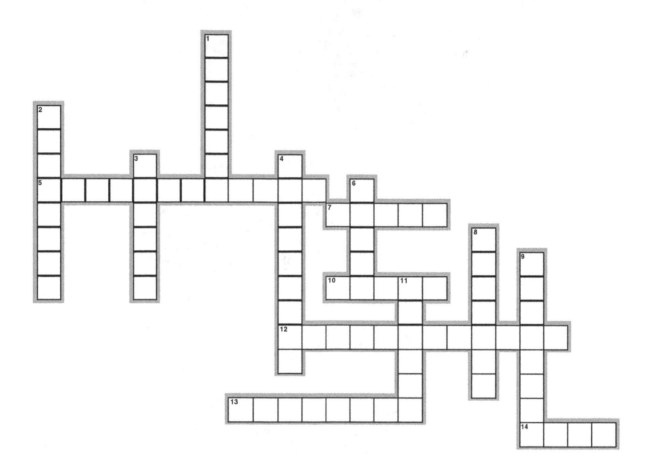

Across

5. Law that states total energy does not change; Law of _____ of Energy
7. British unit for weight or force
10. SI unit for length
12. Change in velocity over time
13. *d/t*
14. Quantity of matter in an object; does not change

Down

1. Property of objects to resist changes in their motion
2. Newton's third law: Action-_____
3. SI Unit for force
4. Energy of position: _____ energy
6. Unit of measurement for work or energy
8. Energy of motion: _____ energy
9. SI unit for mass
11. Ability to do work

Atomic Structure

1. Whose atomic model is used the most frequently to illustrate its structure and demonstrate ionization interactions?

   a. J.J. Thompson
   b. John Dalton
   c. Niels Bohr
   d. Ernest Rutherford

2. Which of the following statements is true regarding atoms?

   a. an atom is mostly empty space
   b. atoms have a net positive charge
   c. all atoms are made of earth, water, fire, and air
   d. an atom has no mass and no charge

3. The Z# is the number of _____ in the nucleus.

   a. protons
   b. neutrons
   c. protons and electrons
   d. protons and neutrons

4. An element with an atomic number of 92 and an atomic mass number of 238 would have:

   a. 92 protons, 146 neutrons, and 92 electrons
   b. 92 protons, 146 neutrons, and 238 electrons
   c. 92 protons, 238 neutrons, and 146 electrons
   d. 146 protons, 92 neutrons, and 92 electrons

5. According to the octet rule:

   a. there are eight possible configurations for Bohr's orbital shell models
   b. there are eight groups in the periodic chart
   c. any atom with an atomic number divisible by eight is unstable
   d. the maximum number of electrons an outer orbital shell can hold is eight

6. The fundamental force that keeps an atom's electrons orbiting the nucleus is:

   a. gravity
   b. electrostatic
   c. gluons
   d. electromagnetic

7. Which of the following is a molecule, rather than an element?

   a. sodium chloride
   b. barium
   c. copper
   d. rubidium

8. A charged atom or an atom with fewer electrons than protons is termed a/an:

   a. positron
   b. negatron
   c. ion
   d. isotope

9. If one electron is taken away from a helium atom, the result is:

   a. hydrogen
   b. an isotope
   c. an ion
   d. radioactive

10. The letter designation for the fourth shell out from the nucleus is:

    a. D
    b. K
    c. L
    d. N

11. The maximum number of electrons that the P orbital shell can theoretically hold is:

    a. 2
    b. 8
    c. 36
    d. 72

12. Sodium, potassium, lithium, and cesium are placed in the same group in the periodic table because they:

    a. contain the same number of protons
    b. share similar chemical properties
    c. have identical atomic mass numbers
    d. are all radioactive elements

13. The general term for the two subatomic particles that occupy the massive, central structure of the atom is:

    a. nucleus
    b. nucleon
    c. proton
    d. neutron

14. The binding energy of a K-shell electron in a tungsten atom is:

    a. 184 keV
    b. 74 keV
    c. 69.5 keV
    d. 37.4 keV

15. Which of the following best describes a proton?

    a. a subatomic particle with a mass of 1 amu and a positive charge
    b. a form of electromagnetic radiation
    c. a subatomic particle with a mass of 1/2,000 amu and a negative charge
    d. an atom with the same number of neutrons and electrons

16. The chemical symbol for the element barium is:

    a. B
    b. Ba
    c. Be
    d. Bm

17. Which of the following elements has the highest Z number?

    a. hydrogen
    b. aluminum
    c. lead
    d. uranium

18. Which of the following information items can be found in each cell of the periodic table?

    1. Atomic number
    2. Atomic weight
    3. Atomic charge

    a. 1, 2
    b. 1, 3
    c. 2, 3
    d. 1, 2, 3

19. The unit commonly used to measure the mass of an atom is the:

    a. gram
    b. amu
    c. pound
    d. joule

20. The atoms, C-12 and C-14, would be classified as:

    a. isotopes
    b. isobars
    c. isotones
    d. isomers

21. Atoms may combine to form molecules by which of the following chemical bonds?

    1. Covalent
    2. Nuclear
    3. Ionic

    a. 1, 2
    b. 1, 3
    c. 2, 3
    d. 1, 2, 3

22. The spontaneous transformation of one element due to the emission of electromagnetic or particulate radiation is the definition for:

    a. energy
    b. half-life
    c. radioactivity
    d. ionization

23. The type(s) of electromagnetic radiation emitted by a radioisotope is/are:

    1. Alpha
    2. Beta
    3. Gamma

    a. 1 only
    b. 3 only
    c. 1, 2
    d. 1, 2, 3

24. How many half-lives will it take for an isotope (e.g., 100 mCi Tc-99m) to decay to <10% (<10 mCi) of its original activity?

    a. 1
    b. 2
    c. 3
    d. 4

25. Which of the following is true regarding radioisotope half-lives?

    a. each radioisotope has a unique half-life
    b. all radioisotopes of the same element have the same half-life
    c. the half-life of each radioisotope gets progressively longer over time
    d. half-life is dependent on whether alpha, beta, and/or gamma radiation(s) are emitted

26. The two types of ionizing radiations that are the most similar in nature are:

    a. x-rays and beta
    b. alpha and gamma
    c. alpha and x-rays
    d. x-rays and gamma

27. Which of the following ionizing radiations has only one unit of negative charge?

    a. gamma rays
    b. beta particle
    c. x-rays
    d. alpha particle

28. Alpha decay is characterized by:

    a. A # decreased by 4, Z# decreased by 2
    b. A # increased by 4, Z# increased by 2
    c. A # remains stable, Z# increased by 1
    d. A # increased by 1, Z# increased by 1

29. Select the pair of atoms that are isobars:

    a. I-121 and I-121
    b. I-131 and Xe-131
    c. H-2 and H-2
    d. I-130 and Cs-132

30. Which of the following elements is usually considered radioactive?

    a. technetium
    b. carbon
    c. lead
    d. barium

Image Labeling

1. Identify the subatomic particles and electron shells as indicated in the diagram below.

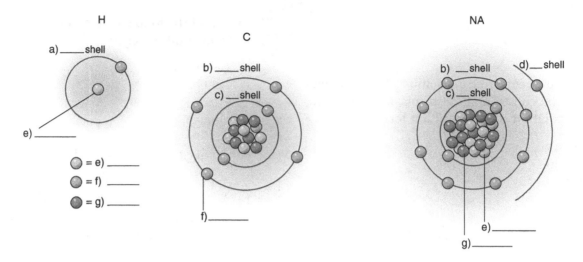

2. Complete the table of atomic mass and charge as indicated.

Particle	Mass in kg	Mass in amu	Charge
Proton	1.6726×10^{-27}	____	_____
Neutron	1.6749×10^{-27}	____	_____
Electron	9.109×10^{-31}	____	_____

3. Label the components of the tungsten atom as indicated.

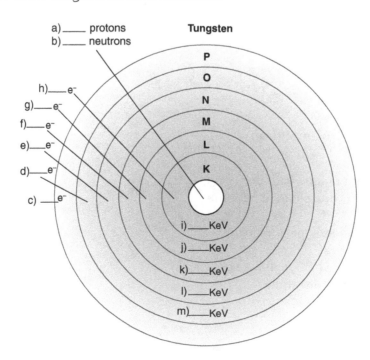

4. Complete the information that can be found in each cell of the periodic table.

a) _____

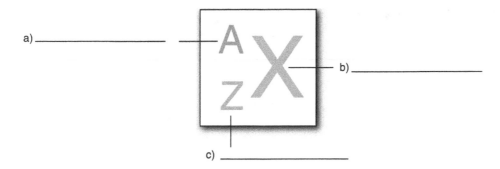

b) _____

c) _____

Crossword Puzzle

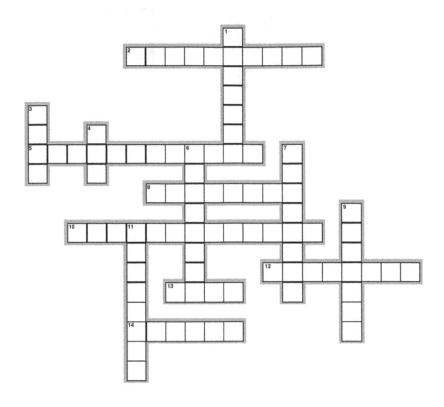

Across

2. Process of adding or removing electrons from an atom
5. Equal to the number of protons in an atom (two words)
8. Time required for a radioisotope to decay to one-half of its initial activity
10. Spontaneous transformation of one element to another due to an unstable nucleus
12. Type of molecular bond when two atoms share an electron orbital
13. Emitted from a radioisotope; equivalent to an electron
14. A nucleon with a positive charge

Down

1. Outer electron shell; determines an atom's ability to combine with another atom
3. The chemical symbol for this element is Pb
4. Atomic mass unit
6. Two or more atoms that are chemically combined, for example, NaCl
7. Has an atomic mass of 1/2,000 amu
9. The positively charged center of an atom
11. Elements with the same number of protons but different numbers of neutrons

Electromagnetic Radiation

5

1. The number of wave cycles per second is the definition for:

   a. wavelength
   b. amplitude
   c. frequency
   d. intensity

2. The distance between the same portions of adjacent waves is the:

   a. wavelength
   b. amplitude
   c. frequency
   d. intensity

3. The variations between zero and maximum height of the wave is the:

   a. wavelength
   b. amplitude
   c. frequency
   d. intensity

4. Hertz is a measure of:

   a. the number of cycles per millimeter
   b. the number of cycles per second
   c. energy per centimeter square
   d. intensity per millimeter

5. One hertz is:

   a. 1 cycle per second
   b. 1,000 cycles per second
   c. 10,000 cycles per second
   d. 1,000,000 cycles per second

6. One kilohertz is:

   a. 1 cycle per second
   b. 1,000 cycles per second
   c. 10,000 cycles per second
   d. 1,000,000 cycles per second

7. Which of the following is not a form of electromagnetic radiation?

   a. microwaves
   b. ultrasound
   c. infrared
   d. x-rays

8. Light travels at a speed of:

   a. 340 mi/s
   b. 10,000 m/s
   c. 3×10^8 m/s
   d. 2.54×10^{18} ft/s

9. Electromagnetic radiation travels in packets of energy called:

   a. photons
   b. protons
   c. rays
   d. Coulombs

10. Which of the following is NOT true regarding electromagnetic radiation?

    a. electromagnetic photons have no mass
    b. photons have varying frequencies and wavelengths
    c. all photons in the electromagnetic spectrum are electrically neutral
    d. alpha and beta radiation have wavelengths slightly longer than gamma

11. If a light signal and a radio signal were emitted simultaneously from Alpha Centauri, a distant star, the first to reach the earth would be the:

    a. radio signal
    b. light signal
    c. both would reach earth at the same time

12. Because the speed of light is constant, an increase in frequency results in _____ in wavelength:

    a. an increase
    b. a decrease
    c. no change

13. All electromagnetic waves have what characteristic in common?

    a. they share the same wavelength
    b. they have the same energy
    c. they all have the same frequency
    d. they all travel at c

14. Which of the following devices emits ultraviolet radiation?

    a. toaster ovens
    b. cell phone towers
    c. tanning beds
    d. airport baggage screeners

15. The lowest energy of visible light is:

    a. red
    b. black
    c. violet
    d. green

16. Place the following electromagnetic waves in order of increasing wavelength:

    1. Visible light
    2. Radio waves
    3. Gamma rays
    4. Infrared

    a. 3, 1, 4, 2
    b. 4, 1, 2, 3
    c. 2, 4, 1, 3
    d. 3, 4, 1, 2

17. Place the following electromagnetic waves in order of increasing energy:

    1. X-rays
    2. Microwaves
    3. Visible light
    4. Radio

    a. 1, 2, 3, 4
    b. 4, 2, 3, 1
    c. 1, 2, 4, 3
    d. 4, 3, 2, 1

18. Identify the EM radiation below with the highest frequency.

    a. visible light
    b. microwaves
    c. generated AC electricity
    d. ultraviolet

19. Which of the following electromagnetic waves has the longest wavelength?

    a. radio waves
    b. infrared waves
    c. x-rays
    d. ultraviolet waves

20. Which of the following statements best describes the relationship between frequency, wavelength, and energy?

    a. as energy increases, both wavelength and frequency increase
    b. as energy increases, both wavelength and frequency decrease
    c. as energy increases, wavelength increases and frequency decreases
    d. as energy increases, wavelength decreases and frequency increases

21. Using the formula, $E = hf$, calculate the energy of an x-ray photon if its frequency is 1.26×10^{19} Hz:

    a. 6.7×10^{12} keV
    b. 5.2×10^{4} eV
    c. 3.9×10^{-2} J
    d. 8.3×10 eV

22. Using the formula, $c = f\lambda$, calculate the frequency of an x-ray photon that has a wavelength of 2.3×10^{-10} m.

    a. 3×10^{8} m/s
    b. 6.9×10^{-2} Hz
    c. 1.3×10^{18} Hz
    d. 7.6×10^{-17} m

23. Using the formula, $c = f\lambda$, calculate the wavelength of an x-ray photon that has a frequency of 3.28×10^{17} Hz.

    a. 1.09×10^{9} m
    b. 9.84×10^{25} m
    c. 3×10^{8} m/s
    d. 9.15×10^{-10} m

24. The wave-particle duality theory states that:

    a. every point on a light wave converges to a particle
    b. photons can be characterized as particles or a wave
    c. for every electric wave, there is a magnetic wave 90 degree to it
    d. x-rays and gamma rays are identical except for their source

25. Ionizing radiation is radiation that:

    a. is continuously emitted from an MRI unit
    b. has enough energy to remove an electron from its orbital shell
    c. is created using ultrasound
    d. causes charge to be transferred through induction

26. According to the inverse square law, the intensity of radiation:

    a. increases with increasing distance
    b. remains constant at any given distance
    c. decreases with the square of the distance
    d. converges to a point when the distance is squared

27. Based on inverse square law principles, if a technologist is standing 1 m from a radiation source, the intensity she/he will receive if she/he steps back to a distance of 3 m will:

    a. increase
    b. decrease
    c. not change

28. If the original exposure rate to a technologist is 8 mR/h at a distance of 4 m, moving to a distance of 2 m results in a new exposure rate of:

    a. 2 mR/h
    b. 4 mR/h
    c. 16 mR/h
    d. 32 mR/h

29. Calculate the original intensity given the following factors:

    $I_2 = 270$ mR
    $d_1 = 40''$
    $d_2 = 72''$
    $I_1 = $ _____

    a. 83 mR
    b. 150 mR
    c. 486 mR
    d. 875 mR

30. Calculate the new distance given the following factors:

    $I^1 = 26$ mR
    $I^2 = 295$ mR
    $d^1 = 300$ cm
    $d^2 = $ _____

    a. 30 cm
    b. 89 cm
    c. 600 cm
    d. 1,000 cm

Labeling

1. Label the identified parts of the wave

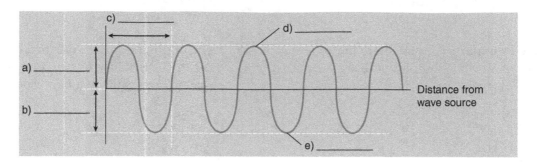

2. Label the identified parts of the wave

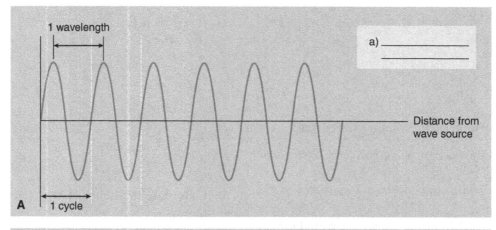

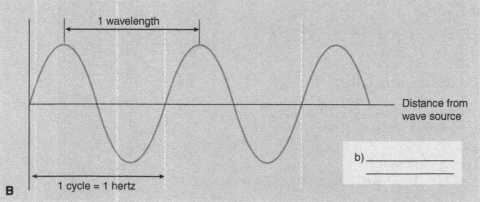

3. Identify the representative portions of the electromagnetic spectrum identified by the letters below in the order of their increasing energy.

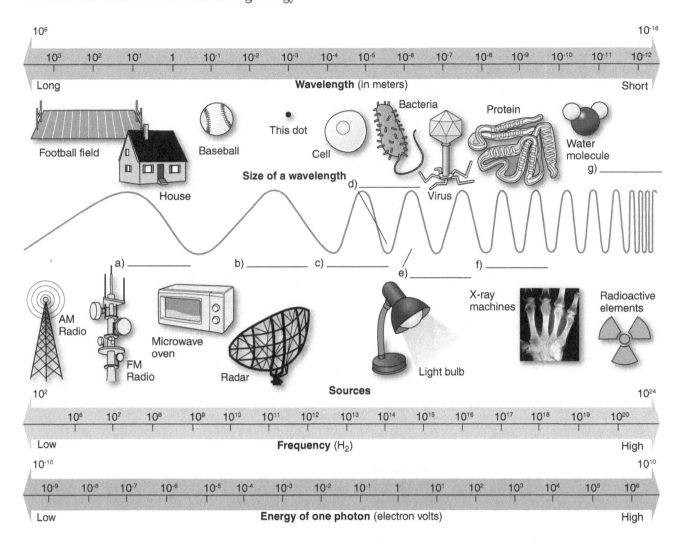

Crossword Puzzle

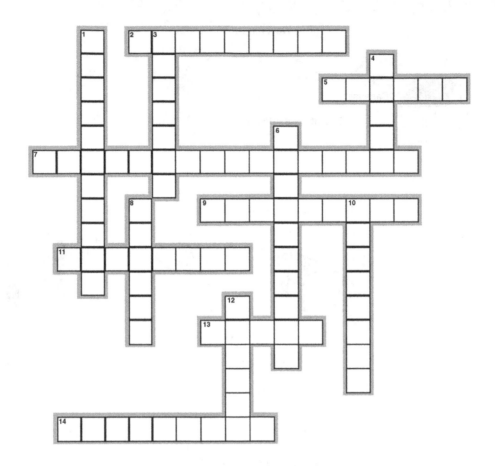

Across

2. Electromagnetic wave that can be used to cook food rapidly
5. German physicist who described the direct relationship between frequency and energy of waves in the formula: $E = hf$
7. States that the intensity of the radiation is inversely proportional to the square of the distance (three words)
9. The flux of energy flow per second; measured in watts/cm^2
11. The speed of a wave
13. Unit that measures the frequency of a wave
14. The magnitude of a wave

Down

1. The electromagnetic wave that falls between visible light and x-rays
3. The relationship between the wavelength and frequency of transverse waves
4. The portion of the electromagnetic spectrum with the shortest wavelength
6. The distance between adjacent peaks or adjacent valleys of a wave
8. A discrete packet of electromagnetic energy
10. Heat energy
12. The time required for one complete cycle of a wave

PART II

Creating the X-Ray Beam

Electricity

1. The four types of electrical materials are:

   a. conductors, inflectors, semiconductors, and superconductors
   b. conductors, insulators, semiconductors, and superconductors
   c. convectors, insulators, semiconductors, and supercollectors
   d. conductors, informers, semicolliders, and superconvectors

2. The unit of electrical potential is the:

   a. watt
   b. ampere
   c. volt
   d. ohm

3. What type of material would be the best insulator?

   a. copper
   b. silver
   c. tap water
   d. glass

4. A superconductor must be _____ to maintain its superconductivity.

   a. cooled
   b. heated
   c. magnetized
   d. energized

5. Increasing the resistance in a circuit results in a(n):

   a. increase in current
   b. increase in voltage
   c. decrease in current
   d. decrease in voltage

6. A charge of 30 C passes at a steady rate through a resistor in a time of 5 s. What is the current through the resistor?

   a. $0.17 \, \Omega$
   b. 3.0 V
   c. 6.0 A
   d. 150 W

7. Which of the following situations would serve to increase the resistance of a wire?

   a. reducing the temperature
   b. doubling the diameter
   c. doubling the length
   d. reducing the distance

8. The equation, $R = V/I$, is used to express:

   a. magnetic flux
   b. Ohm's law
   c. power law
   d. conservation law

9. If a current of 0.5 A flows through a conductor and has a resistance of 6 ohms, the voltage is:

   a. 3 A
   b. 12 V
   c. 3 V
   d. 6.5 W

10. The current through a 5 ohm resistor connected to a 220 V outlet is:

    a. 220 V
    b. 44 A
    c. 1100 A
    d. 5 Ω

11. What is the power rating of a lamp that carries 2 A at 120 V?

    a. 120 W
    b. 60 W
    c. 0.167 W
    d. 240 W

12. Voltage can be induced in a wire by:

    a. moving a magnet near the wire
    b. placing the south pole of a magnet near the north pole of another magnet
    c. rubbing magnets together
    d. connecting it to a galvanometer

13. The force needed to pass a current of one ampere through a resistance of one ohm is the definition for the:

    a. volt
    b. work
    c. ampere
    d. watt

14. Amperage is used to define:

    a. the direction of flow of electrons through a conductor
    b. the electromotive force impressed on the conductor
    c. the resistance offered by the flow of electricity
    d. a Coulomb of charge passing a given point in one second

15. An excessive amount of electrons at one end of a conductor and a deficiency at the other end is known as:

    a. space charge
    b. resistance
    c. potential difference
    d. impedance

16. In a 60-cycle alternating current, how many complete cycles are there every second?

    a. 30
    b. 60
    c. 120
    d. 180

17. Electric insulators:

    a. store electric charge
    b. permit the movement of electric charge
    c. inhibit the movement of electric charge
    d. change electric charges from positive to negative

18. The unit of electrical power is the:

    a. ohm
    b. volt
    c. ampere
    d. watt

19. The normal flow of electrons in an x-ray tube is from a _____ cathode to a _____ anode.

    a. negative; positive
    b. positive; negative
    c. cold; hot
    d. magnetic south; magnetic north

20. Electrification occurs when:

    a. hydrogen atoms align in the presence of a magnet
    b. electrons are transferred through direct contact
    c. positively charged protons are converted to negatively charged electrons
    d. a charge is transferred by grounding

21. The unit of the charge is the _____ with a value of:

    a. electron; 1.6×10^{-19} C
    b. ohm; 1 V/I
    c. coulomb; 6.3×10^{18} electrons
    d. watt; 1 J/s

22. According to the Laws of Electrostatics, which of the following statements is true?

    a. a positive charge and a negative charge will be attracted to each other
    b. charge resides in the center of the conductor
    c. the force of the attraction-repulsion between two charges is directly proportional to the distance between them
    d. electrostatic charge concentration is greatest in spheres

23. In order for current to flow:

    a. a vacuum must be created
    b. a potential difference must exist
    c. a superconductor must be heated
    d. charge must be aligned with the direction of gravity

24. What four components are required for a basic electrical circuit?

    a. alternating current, anode, cathode, and a vacuum tube
    b. conductor, switch, load/resistor, and a power/voltage source
    c. watts, volts, amps, and ohms
    d. direct current, alternating current, a large diameter wire, and high temperatures

25. Two 15-ohm resistances are connected in series with one another. What is the total resistance of this circuit?

    a. 0.13 ohms
    b. 7.5 ohms
    c. 15 ohms
    d. 30 ohms

26. The primary advantage of a parallel circuit is that:

    a. as more appliances are added less current is used
    b. as more appliances are added, each appliance receives less voltage
    c. failure of one appliance does NOT prevent the operation of others in the circuit
    d. it is the simplest type of circuit

27. When more resistors are added in a PARALLEL circuit, which statement below is true?

    a. the total voltage of the circuit is decreased
    b. the total voltage of the circuit is increased
    c. the total resistance is decreased
    d. the total resistance is increased

28. What is the total resistance of a 10-ohm, 500-ohm, 1,000-ohm, 5,000-ohm, and a 100,000-ohm connected in parallel?

    a. 16,500-ohms
    b. greater than 500 ohms but less than 10,000-ohms
    c. greater than 100,000-ohms
    d. greater than 10-ohms
    e. less than 10-ohms

29. Three resistances of 4, 6, and 12 ohms, respectively, are connected in parallel. What is their combined resistance?

    a. 0.5 ohms
    b. 1.64 ohms
    c. 2 ohms
    d. 22 ohms

30. Which of the following rules applies to series circuits?

    a. $V_T = V_1 = V_2 = V_3 \ldots$
    b. $R_T = R_1 + R_2 + R_3 \ldots$
    c. $1/R_T = 1/R_1 + 1/R_2 + 1/R_3 \ldots$
    d. $I_T = I_1 + I_2 + I_3 \ldots$

Labeling

1. Analyze the conductor illustration shown. For lines a and b, indicate which arrow is actual electron flow and which is conventional current flow.

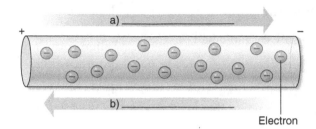

2. Complete the table describing the four types of electrical materials.

Type of Material	Characteristics	Examples
Conductor		
Insulator		
Semiconductor		
Superconductor		

3. Label the components of the electric circuit shown.

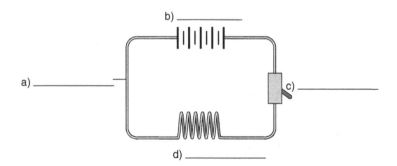

4. Identify each circuit type shown. In the space provided, write the equation used to calculate total resistance in each circuit

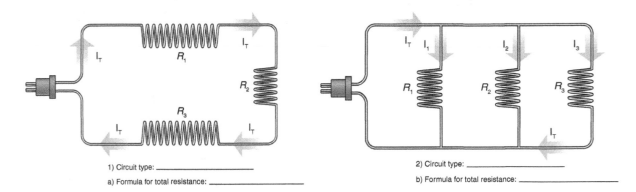

1) Circuit type: _____

a) Formula for total resistance: _____

2) Circuit type: _____

b) Formula for total resistance: _____

Crossword Puzzle

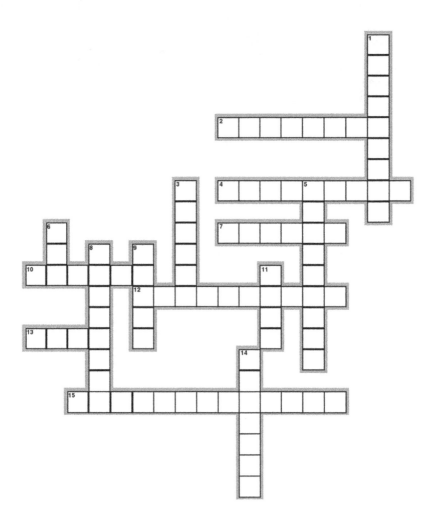

Across

2. Type of circuit where the level of voltage in each branch is equal to the total voltage
4. A method of charging a neutral object without actual contact
7. A charge object is neutralized when it is directed to the _____.
10. Unit to measure current
12. Electrical property that opposes current flow
13. Unit used to measure electrical potential difference
15. Rectifiers in an x-ray circuit are made from this type of material

Down

1. Material where electrons are held tightly in place
3. Type of circuit where all the elements are connected in one path
5. Material that allows electrons to move freely
6. The unit for electrical resistance
8. Actual direction of electron flow; from _____ to positive
9. Unit to measure alternating current's frequency; equal to one cycle per second
11. Unit used to measure power
14. Unit of charge

Electromagnetism

7

1. The units of magnetism are the:

   a. grass and tesla
   b. gauss and tesly
   c. gruss and tesly
   d. gauss and tesla

2. Which of these materials is not ferromagnetic?

   a. iron
   b. wood
   c. nickel
   d. cobalt

3. Which of these materials is ferromagnetic?

   a. wood
   b. glass
   c. iron
   d. plastic

4. A ferromagnetic material is:

   a. weakly influenced by a magnetic field
   b. strongly influenced by a magnetic field
   c. repelled by a magnetic field
   d. not influenced at all

5. Two magnets with the same poles facing each other will:

   a. be attracted
   b. be repelled
   c. experience a force times the distance
   d. experience no force

6. When a charged particle is put in motion:

   a. a magnetic field is created
   b. an electric dipole has been ionized
   c. gamma radiation results
   d. it allows positive charges in a conductor to move, also

7. According to electromagnetic induction principles, which of the following situations will serve to increase the amount of voltage produced?

   a. increasing the number of loops in the wire
   b. changing the motion of the magnet from 90 degrees to parallel
   c. stopping the motion of the magnet
   d. slowing the motion of the coil

8. An electric motor converts:

   a. mechanical energy to electrical energy
   b. electrical energy to mechanical energy
   c. electrical energy to chemical energy
   d. chemical energy to electrical energy

9. The core of an electromagnet should be made of:

   a. silver
   b. iron
   c. tungsten
   d. copper

10. **A coiled helix carrying an electric current is known as a:**

    a. generator
    b. rectifier
    c. transformer
    d. solenoid

11. **Mechanical energy can be converted into electrical energy by a:**

    a. capacitor
    b. generator
    c. battery
    d. motor

12. **A changing magnetic field produces:**

    a. insulation
    b. sound waves
    c. an electric field
    d. electromagnetic radiation

13. **Maximum induction will occur when a conductor cuts a magnetic field at what angle?**

    a. 0 degrees
    b. 45 degrees
    c. 90 degrees
    d. 180 degrees

14. **A solenoid with an iron core in its center is called a/n:**

    a. motor
    b. alternator
    c. generator
    d. electromagnet

15. **What type of motor drives the rotating anode in the x-ray tube?**

    a. synchronous
    b. induction
    c. direct current
    d. inductive reactance

16. **A simple DC generator is similar to an AC generator except that a DC generator is constructed with:**

    a. an armature
    b. slip rings
    c. commutator
    d. brushes

17. **During the process of mutual induction:**

    a. electron flow is impeded
    b. current flows in only one direction
    c. current is transferred from one coil to another
    d. a semiconductor becomes magnetized

18. **In his experiments in 1820, Hans Christian Oersted, a Danish physicist, concluded that:**

    a. electricity and magnetism were in no way related
    b. electricity and magnetism must be related forces
    c. magnetism is increased in the presence of resistors
    d. a compass could be used to conduct electricity

19. **Michael Faraday discovered electromagnetic induction. He proved that voltage can be induced in a wire by:**

    a. connecting it to a galvanometer
    b. moving a magnet near the wire
    c. placing the south pole of a magnet near the north pole of another magnet
    d. rubbing magnets together

20. **The purpose of adding an iron core to a solenoid is to:**

    a. increase the strength of the magnetic field
    b. impede the path of the electrons
    c. allow voltage and current to be changed independently
    d. boil off more electrons during thermionic emission

21. **Generators, motors, and transformers all operate due to this principle:**

    a. inverse square law
    b. Coulomb's Law
    c. Ohm's Law
    d. electromagnetic induction

22. **A primary difference between electrostatic charges and magnetic poles are that:**

    a. only electrical charges have a definable field surrounding them
    b. the repulsion-attraction laws governing them are opposite for each
    c. electrostatic charges can be isolated, while magnetic poles cannot
    d. a magnetic field cannot be used to generate electricity, while electrostatic charges can

23. **Lodestone is another name for:**

    a. a superconductor
    b. a natural magnet
    c. an alloy of aluminum, cobalt, and nickel
    d. a temporary magnet

24. **Which of the following situations are capable of producing a magnetic domain?**

    1. A current-carrying wire
    2. An MRI unit
    3. Replacing a copper conductor with plastic

    a. 1, 2
    b. 1, 3
    c. 2, 3
    d. 1, 2, 3

25. **According to the Inverse Square Law, which governs all electrical and magnetic waves, if the distance from the source of radiation is decreased by two times, the intensity will:**

    a. increase by four times
    b. decrease by four times
    c. increase by eight times
    d. decrease by eight times

26. **According to Lenz's law, the induced EMF in a coil:**

    a. creates a current in the opposite direction
    b. is inverse to the frequency of the motion
    c. always creates a north magnetic pole
    d. produces direct current

27. **In order for self-induction and mutual induction to occur,**

    a. the commutator ring must be grounded
    b. a DC generator must be used to power the circuit
    c. the rotor must consist of copper and iron outside a vacuum tube
    d. a continuously changing magnetic field must be produced

28. **An application of an induction motor is used in the x-ray tube to:**

    a. power the rotating anode
    b. generate thermionic emission
    c. run the cooling fans
    d. provide electricity for the light field in the collimator

29. **Which of the following x-ray tube components contains an even number of stationary electromagnets that induce current into copper bars through the use of AC?**

    a. anode
    b. stator
    c. rotor
    d. filament

30. **The x-ray circuit component that works using self-induction is the:**

    a. anode
    b. high voltage transformer
    c. autotransformer
    d. high voltage resistor

Labeling

1. Analyze the magnetic poles below and complete each label, indicating whether it attracts or repels. Also add arrows to indicate the direction of the magnetic force between the two poles.

a) _____

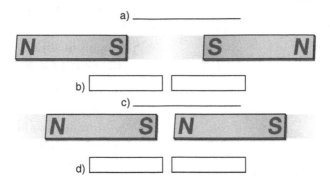

b)   [_____]   [_____]

c) _____

d)   [_____]   [_____]

2. Label the electrical components shown.

Single turn on coil

a) _____

A

Many turns on coil

+ terminal

b) _____

− terminal

B

Ferromagnetic core added

+ terminal

c) _____

− terminal

C

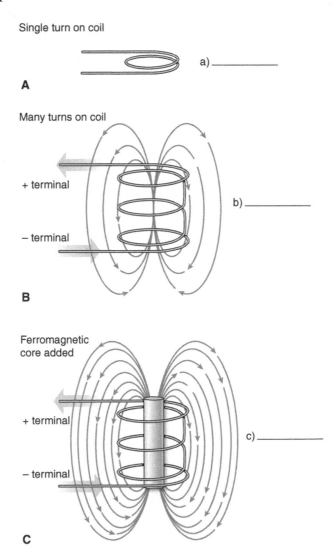

3. Label the components of the mutual induction process.

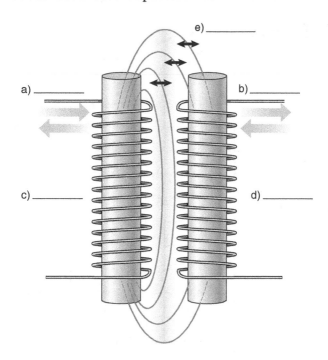

e) _____

a) _____   b) _____

c) _____   d) _____

4. Identify the parts of an AC induction motor.

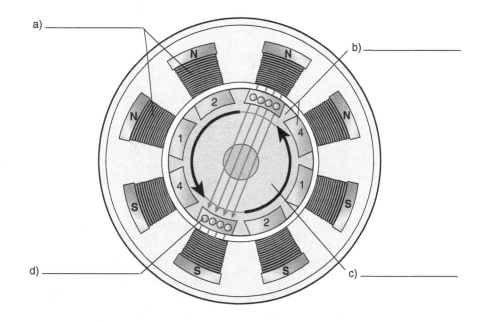

a) _____   b) _____

d) _____   c) _____

Crossword Puzzle

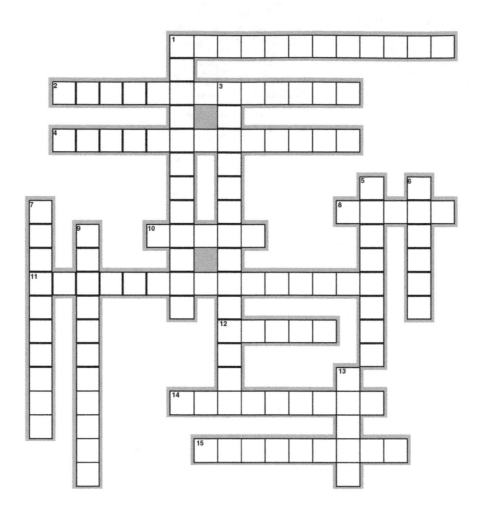

Across

1. Ability of a material to be magnetized
2. A device that contains an iron core in a coiled conductor; a mechanism used to produce current
4. Materials that are attracted to a magnet
8. The _____ pole of a magnet would be attracted to the south pole of another magnet
10. A single coil of a conducting material
11. Occurs when two coils are placed next to each other; allows current to be transferred to each other without touching (two words)
12. Electromagnetic device that converts electrical energy into mechanical energy
14. Electromagnetic device that converts mechanical energy into electrical energy
15. A natural magnet

Down

1. Material that displays a weak attraction to magnetic fields; gadolinium is an example
3. Group of atoms whose dipoles are aligned in the same direction (two words)
5. A coiled conductor with an iron core
6. Electrical component outside the glass envelope of an x-ray tube; contains stationary electromagnets to cause the rotor to turn
7. Type of ring used in a DC generator instead of a slip ring
9. Ability of a magnet to retain its magnetic properties
13. Causes the anode to spin in an x-ray tube, consists of copper bars around an iron core

8

X-Ray Unit Circuitry

1. The component of an x-ray circuit that maintains a consistent level of voltage to the x-ray circuit is the/a:

   a. generator
   b. step-up transformer
   c. rheostat
   d. line voltage compensator

2. A transformer with 300 turns on the primary side, input side and 40,000 turns on the secondary side is a _____ transformer

   a. step-up
   b. step-down
   c. autotransformer
   d. shell type

3. A transformer with more turns on the secondary windings than the primary windings would be expected to:

   a. increase the voltage and decrease the amperage
   b. increase the voltage and increase the amperage
   c. decrease the voltage and decrease the amperage
   d. decrease the voltage and increase the amperage

4. The step-up transformer in an x-ray circuit:

   a. has six moving parts
   b. requires DC to induce a current
   c. requires AC for mutual inductance to occur
   d. operates on both DC and AC

5. What effect(s) does a step-down transformer have on current and voltage?

   1. Current increases
   2. Current decreases
   3. Voltage increases
   4. Voltage decreases
   5. Current remains constant
   6. Voltage remains constant

   a. 1, 6
   b. 3, 5
   c. 5, 4
   d. 1, 4

6. A transformer has 200,000 turns in the primary and 50,000 turns in the secondary. The turns ratio of this transformer is:

   a. 0.25
   b. 250
   c. 4
   d. 150

7. If a transformer has 200 turns in the primary and 600 turns in the secondary and the input voltage is 110 volts, the output voltage for this transformer would be:

   a. 3 volts
   b. 36.7 volts
   c. 220 volts
   d. 330 volts

8. Which of the following transformer types is designed with a central iron core wrapped with both the primary and secondary windings to promote maximum mutual induction?

    a. open core transformer
    b. autotransformer
    c. closed core transformer
    d. shell type transformer

9. The selection of the kVp for an x-ray exposure is made by changing which component of the x-ray circuit?

    a. rheostat
    b. rectifier
    c. cathode
    d. autotransformer

10. The electronic timer used in most contemporary x-ray circuits today uses what preprogrammed electrical device to store charge and terminate the exposure?

    a. rheostat
    b. switch
    c. capacitor
    d. an ionization chamber

11. A step-down transformer is used in the filament current to change the incoming voltage and current to which of the following ranges?

    a. 5 to 15 volts and 3 to 5 amperes
    b. 100 to 110 volts and 60 to 100 amperes
    c. 110 to 220 volts and 110 to 220 amperes
    d. 50 to 120 kilovolts and 25 to 1,200 milliamperes

12. The component in an x-ray circuit which is responsible for varying current is a:

    a. rheostat
    b. capacitor
    c. transformer
    d. rectifier

13. When it is necessary to change alternating current to direct current, _____ are placed into the circuit.

    a. rheostats
    b. high voltage transformers
    c. rectifiers
    d. ammeters

14 to 24. In Questions 14 through 24, match the component of the x-ray circuit with its description.

14. _____ Autotransformer
15. _____ Rectifiers
16. _____ Anode
17. _____ kVp meter
18. _____ Glass envelope
19. _____ Step-down transformer
20. _____ Step-up transformer
21. _____ Filament
22. _____ Cathode
23. _____ Rotor
24. _____ mA meter

a. Negative side of the x-ray tube
b. Measures the EMF in the circuit
c. Converts alternating current to direct current
d. Adjusts voltage downward
e. Source of electrons
f. Positive side of the x-ray tube
g. Contains only one coil; serves as kVp selector
h. Converts voltage to the kilovoltage range
i. Serves to rotate the anode
j. Provides a vacuum environment
k. Measures current in the secondary circuit

25. Which of the following circuits and type of rectification uses two rectifiers in the x-ray circuit?

    a. single phase, half-wave
    b. single phase, full-wave
    c. three phase, full-wave, 6 pulse
    d. three phase, full-wave, 12 pulse

26. Which type of x-ray circuit would exhibit frequencies in the 500 to 3,000 Hertz range?

    a. single phase, half-wave
    b. single phase, high frequency
    c. three phase, 6 pulse
    d. six phase, 12 pulse

27. Ripple measures

    a. total tube voltage
    b. variation between maximum and minimum mA
    c. variation between maximum and minimum tube voltage
    d. total mA

28. A three-phase, six pulse x-ray circuit would exhibit approximately how much ripple in its voltage waveform?

    a. 4%
    b. 14%
    c. 1%
    d. 100%

29. The ionization detectors that are employed in most automatic exposure controlled units are located between the _____ and the _____.

    a. tube/collimator
    b. collimator/patient
    c. filter/grid
    d. patient/image receptor

30. If an imaging department which utilizes an automatic exposure controlled (AEC) makes a change in its image receptor, what changes must be made for optimum operation of the AEC unit?

    a. all techniques must be doubled
    b. the back-up timer must be inactivated
    c. service should be called to have the AEC recalibrated
    d. detector configurations need to be altered for each exam

31. Which of the following circumstances would cause the back-up timer to activate during the operation of an AEC unit?

    a. a tabletop exam is being performed with the chest board selected
    b. the rectifiers cease functioning causing insufficient current to the tube
    c. an extremely slender or pediatric patient is being examined and the normal detector configurations are chosen.
    d. the technologist has erroneously selected an option to increase the exposure adjustment 30% when it is not necessary

Labeling

1. Label each type of transformer shown.

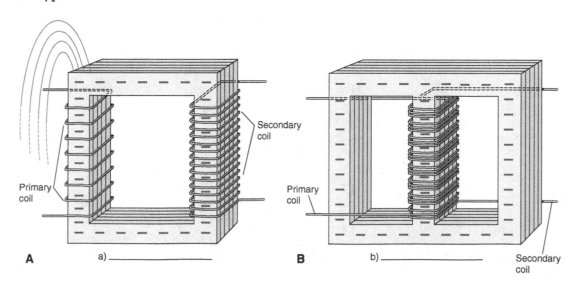

Primary coil

Secondary coil

A   a) _____

Primary coil

B   b) _____   Secondary coil

2. Label the components lettered a through i of the x-ray circuit diagram provided.

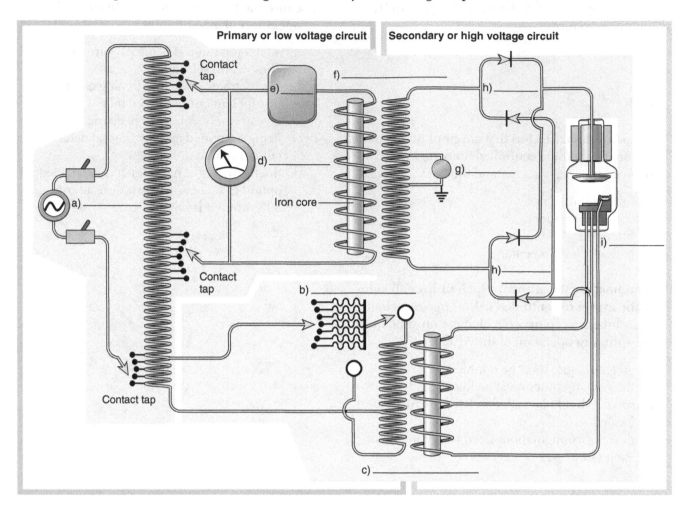

3. Identify each voltage waveform.

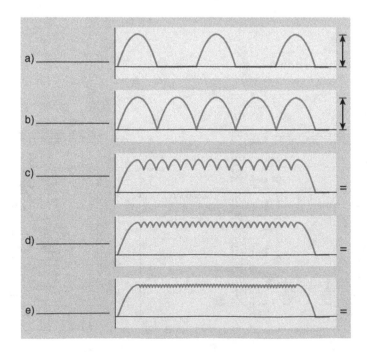

4. For each type of circuit listed, complete the table identifying its maximum percent voltage and its percentage of ripple.

Type of Circuit	Average % of Set kV	Percent Ripple
Single-phase	_____	_____
Three-phase, 6-pulse	_____	_____
Three-phase, 12-pulse	_____	_____
High-frequency generator	_____	_____

Crossword Puzzle

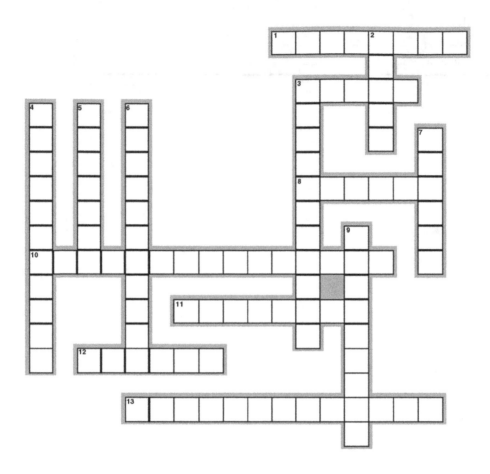

Across

1. Allows resistance to be varied; acts as a milliampere selector for the filament circuit
3. Number of detectors most commonly found in an AEC configuration
8. Type of transformer that would have a voltage output greater than the input
10. A device with a single winding used to step up or down voltage; connected to the kVp selector
11. The step-down transformer is responsible for producing the high current needed for this x-ray tube component
12. Type of current produced by rectifiers
13. Type of x-ray circuit that exhibits only 1% ripple

Down

2. Type of transformer constructed with both primary and secondary winding wrapped around its central iron core
3. Electrical device used to increase or decrease voltage
4. Type of current that transformers require in order to operate
5. In automatic exposure control systems, the detector is placed between the _____ and the image receptor
6. Terminates the exposure in an AEC system before tube limits are exceeded
7. Amount of variation between the maximum and minimum voltage produced in the circuit
9. Device that allows electrons to flow in only one direction; converts AC to DC

The X-Ray Tube

1. The heel effect:

   a. exists because some x-rays are absorbed by the surface of the anode
   b. is caused by the charge difference between the anode and the cathode
   c. depends on the mA and kVp
   d. is reduced by dual focal spots

2. The principle material used in the filament is _____ due to its _____.

   a. lead; ability to stop leakage radiation
   b. aluminum; relatively low cost
   c. nickel; low negative charge
   d. tungsten; high melting point

3. The line focus principle:

   a. makes the focal spot appear larger than it really is
   b. makes use of an angled cathode structure
   c. produces x-ray lines
   d. spreads the heat over a larger part of the anode

4. The purpose of the cathode focusing cup is to:

   a. alter the filament size
   b. group the electrons for their passage to the anode
   c. regulate anode rotation speed
   d. increase the heat capacity of the tube

If the maximum heat load of a tube in a single-phase circuit is 30,000 HU, which of the exposure series in Questions 5 through 9 is permitted on a cold tube? Answer A for allowed or B for not allowed.

5. _____ Five 100 kVp, 300 mA, 0.25 followed by one 100 kVp, 100 mA, 0.1 s exposures

6. _____ Five 120 kVp, 200 mA, 0.2 s exposures

7. _____ Five 80 kVp, 400 mA, 0.2 s exposures

8. _____ Six 75 kVp, 350 mA, 0.2 s exposures

9. _____ Five 80 kVp, 350 mA, 0.2 s exposures

10. A molybdenum shaft is used to connect the anode to the rotor because:

    a. it is a less dense metal with a high melting point
    b. it is easily compressed
    c. it has a high inertia
    d. it produces 17.5 keV x-rays

11. Many x-ray tubes have two filaments:

    a. because the second filament can be used as a spare when the first one burns out
    b. to provide two focal spots
    c. to allow cooling of the filament by alternating exposures
    d. to improve tube cooling by sharing the heat between two filaments

12. The principle means of heat transfer from the anode to the rotor assembly is:

    a. conduction
    b. convection
    c. radiation
    d. induction

13. During the prep portion of an x-ray exposure:

    a. high voltage and x-rays are produced
    b. the filament is deposited on the glass envelope
    c. the anode begins rotating and the filament heats up
    d. the heel effect occurs, resulting in off-focus radiation

In Questions 14 through 16, answer A for true or B for false

14. _____ An increase in target angle will increase the heat capacity of the tube.

15. _____ An increase in focal spot size will increase the heat capacity of the tube.

16. _____ An increase in anode rotation speed will increase the heat capacity of the tube.

The maximum number of heat units allowed per exposure for a high frequency unit is 19,740 HU Based on this maximum value, would the exposures in questions 17 through 21 be safe? Answer A for yes or B for no.

17. _____ 100 mA, 70 kVp, 2 s

18. _____ 400 mA, 60 kVp, 1 s

19. _____ 100 mA, 110 kVp, 1 s

20. _____ 350 mA, 70 kVp, 2 s

21. _____ 200 mA, 80 kVp, 1 s

22. The purpose of the fan in the tube housing is to:

    a. prevent heat buildup on the filament
    b. provide additional kinetic energy to the projectile electrons
    c. ensure that the tube's maximum HU is not exceeded
    d. promote heat dissipation

The effective focal spot will increase with which of the changes or conditions. In questions 23 through 25, answer A for true or B for false.

23. _____ Selecting a larger filament size

24. _____ Increasing the anode angle

25. _____ Increasing the anode rotation speed

26. Which of the following does not improve the heat capacity of the tube?

    a. a rotating anode
    b. an increased target angle
    c. larger focal spots
    d. thermionic emission

27. What are the approximate heat units produced for a high frequency exposure taken at 120 kVp, 300 mA, and 0.6 s?

    a. 21,500
    b. 30,250
    c. 36,000
    d. 86,500

28. Average anode rotation speeds in diagnostic x-ray tubes are in the ranges of:

    a. 3,000 to 10,000 rpm
    b. 200 to 1,200 rpm
    c. 3 to 6 × 10^8 rpm
    d. 1 to 2 rps

29. The heel effect is more pronounced:

    a. with a smaller SID
    b. with a large focal spot
    c. with a large target angle
    d. with a higher speed anode rotation

30. The effective focal spot is determined by the target angle and the:

    a. distance from the anode to cathode
    b. composition of the anode
    c. diameter of the anode
    d. filament size

31. The disadvantage of a small target angle is:

    a. increased heat distribution and capacity
    b. greater field coverage
    c. a greater anode heel effect
    d. more uniform radiographic density

32. Thermionic emission is the emission of:

    a. thermions
    b. electrons from a heated cathode
    c. electrons from a heated anode
    d. x-rays from the tube housing

33. The tube current (mA) is changed by changing the:

    a. filament current
    b. anode voltage
    c. focal spot size
    d. exposure time

34. To extend x-ray tube life, the technologist should:

    1. Perform warm-up exposures at the beginning of each day
    2. Extend the time that the prep button is held down
    3. Avoid repeated exposures at or near the tube's capacity

    a. 1, 2
    b. 1, 3
    c. 2, 3
    d. 1, 2, 3

35. Which chart should be consulted to ensure that adequate time has passed before making additional exposures?

    a. a tube rating chart
    b. an x-ray emission spectrum
    c. an anode cooling curve
    d. a heat unit index

Labeling

1. Label the components of the x-ray tube

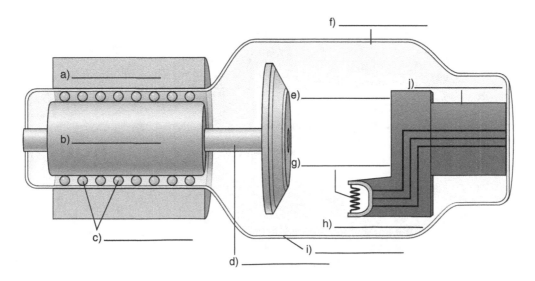

2. **Identify the anode angles and their respective actual and effective focal spots**

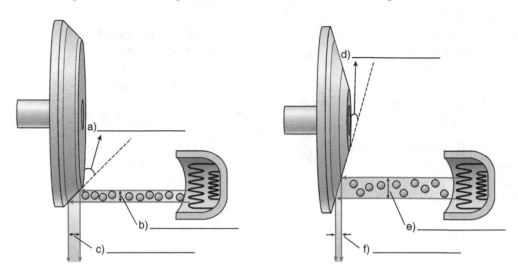

a)_____

b)_____

c)_____

d)_____

e)_____

f)_____

3. **Complete letters a through g below specifying the x-ray intensity range variations caused by the heel effect**

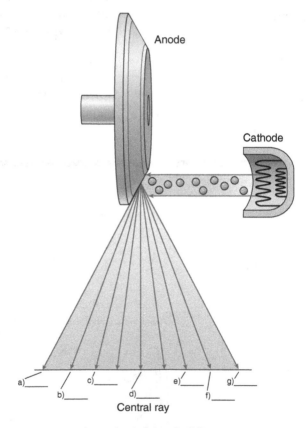

Anode

Cathode

a)____   b)____   c)____   d)____   e)____   f)____   g)____

Central ray

Approximate intensity (%)

Crossword Puzzle

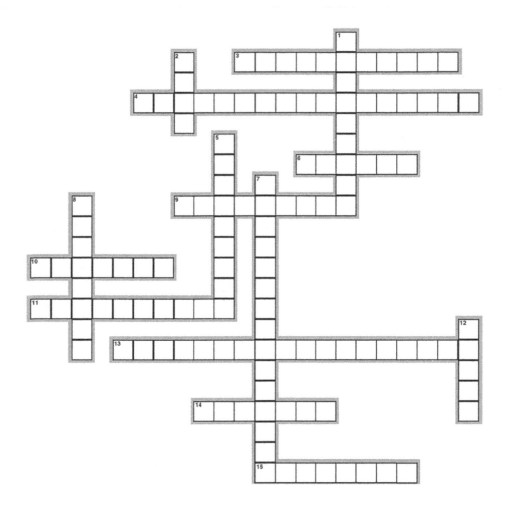

Across

3. Keeps the electron cloud together before they leave the cathode
4. Occurs when no more electrons can be boiled off the filament; limits x-ray tubes to a maximum of 1,000 to 1,200 mA
6. Environment inside the x-ray tube once all air has been removed
9. The product of kVp, mA, and time
10. Type of radiation emitted outside the tube housing; must be less than 100 mR/h at 1 m from the tube
11. Causes uneven distribution of x-ray intensity between the cathode and anode
13. The process of boiling off electrons at the filament
14. The negative electrode of an x-ray tube
15. The anode is constructed of this material due to its high melting point

Down

1. The principle which spreads heat over a greater area of the anode and allows the effective focal spot to be smaller than the actual focal spot
2. 99% of an x-ray tube's output is this form of energy
5. Area where electrons strike the anode
7. Graph which allows radiographers to determine the maximum technical factor combination which is safe for the x-ray tube
8. A coil of wire; source of electrons
12. The positive electrode of an x-ray tube

X-Ray Production

1. Characteristic radiation is produced when:

   a. electrons are stopped at the cathode
   b. a vacancy in an electron orbit is filled
   c. a vacancy in the nucleus is filled
   d. electrons are stopped at the anode

2. X-ray tube filtration filters out:

   a. low-energy electrons
   b. high-energy electrons
   c. low-energy x-rays
   d. high-energy x-rays

3. When an incident electron approaches a positively charged nucleus of a tungsten atom:

   a. the incident electron slows down due to electrostatic attraction
   b. the incident electron penetrates the nucleus
   c. a cascade of electrons from each orbital shell is initiated
   d. a characteristic photon is emitted

4. As kVp is increased, the production of bremsstrahlung photons:

   a. decreases
   b. increases
   c. is replaced by characteristic interactions
   d. remains the same, but lower energy ranges are observed

5. If 90 kVp is selected when a tungsten target is used:

   a. the maximum energy of the projectile electrons and the subsequent x-ray photons will be equal to 30 keV
   b. characteristic photons will be emitted at 30 keV and 90 keV
   c. the kinetic energy of the projectile electrons will be equivalent to this energy and the maximum energy of the x-ray beam will be 90 keV
   d. the projectile energy of the incident photons will be 90 keV and the E_{MAX} of the x-ray beam will be 30 keV

6. In a tungsten target, projectile electrons must have an energy of at least _____ keV to produce K characteristic x-rays.

   a. 50
   b. 70
   c. 67
   d. 58

7. More than _____ percentage of an x-ray beam is made up of photons produced by the bremsstrahlung process.

   a. 1
   b. 10
   c. 80
   d. 90

8. The Cascade process is associated with:

   a. molybdenum targets
   b. brems radiation production
   c. characteristic radiation production
   d. filtration effects

9. Bremsstrahlung produces a _____ energy spectrum.

   a. discrete
   b. continuous
   c. kinetic
   d. filtered

10. Which factors affect characteristic radiation emitted from the x-ray tube?

    a. mA
    b. kVp
    c. filtration
    d. anode material

11. Changing _____ will change the maximum energy of the photons in the x-ray emission spectrum.

    1. mA
    2. kVp
    3. Filtration
    4. Anode material

    a. 1 only
    b. 2 only
    c. 2, 3
    d. 2, 3, 4

12. A technologist can control the quantity of the x-rays striking the patient by adjusting the:

    a. mA
    b. kVp
    c. rectification
    d. anode material

13. The maximum kinetic energy of a projectile electron accelerated across an x-ray tube depends on the:

    a. atomic number Z of the target
    b. size of the focal spot
    c. kilovoltage
    d. type of rectification

14. Beam quality is affected by which of the following factors?

    a. mA
    b. filtration
    c. target angle
    d. focal spot size

15. Beam quantity is primarily determined by:

    a. mAs
    b. kVp
    c. focal spot size
    d. target angle

16. Which of the following types of radiation cannot be produced at tube potentials of less than 70 keV?

    a. bremsstrahlung
    b. scatter
    c. characteristic
    d. primary

17. The process of removing low-energy photons from the x-ray beam is called:

    a. rectification
    b. ionization
    c. electron transition
    d. filtration

18. After electrons strike the anode of an x-ray tube, the majority of the energy is converted to:

    a. heat
    b. bremsstrahlung photons
    c. characteristic photons
    d. kinetic

19. Which of the following can be determined from an x-ray emission spectrum?

    1. Maximum photon energy
    2. Photon velocity
    3. Average photon energy

    a. 1, 2
    b. 1, 3
    c. 2, 3
    d. 1, 2, 3

In Questions 20 through 23, match the x-ray spectrum change with the indicated technique change.

20. _____ mA decreased
21. _____ kVp increased
22. _____ Filtration increased
23. _____ Target Z# decreased

a. Shifts minimum energy of spectrum to the right
b. Causes peaks (amplitude) of graph to decrease
c. Amplitude, maximum and average energy all increased
d. Characteristic radiation appear in new positions

Use the figure below for Questions 24 through 28.

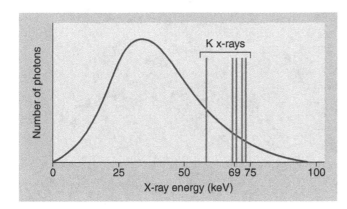

24. The average energy of this beam is approximately _____ keV.

   a. 35
   b. 50
   c. 60
   d. 100

25. The maximum energy of this beam is approximately _____ keV.

   a. 0
   b. 35
   c. 60
   d. 100

26. The energy of the characteristic x-rays is approximately _____ keV.

   a. 0 to 15
   b. 25 to 35
   c. 60 to 70
   d. 90 to 100

27. The applied voltage that produced this beam is approximately _____.

   a. 20 kVp
   b. 40 kVp
   c. 60 kVp
   d. 100 kVp

28. The heterogeneous wavelengths of this x-ray beam is represented by:

   a. the line stretching from 0 to 100 keV
   b. the midpoint of the graph
   c. the spikes shown at approximately 60 and 70 kVp
   d. only the two end points of the graph

29. Which of the following technical factors plays no role in x-ray production?

   a. mA
   b. kVp
   c. time
   d. SID

30. If a projectile electron ionizes a K-shell electron, what x-ray production process has occurred?

   a. bremsstrahlung
   b. characteristic
   c. photoelectric
   d. Compton

Labeling

1. Evaluate the two diagrams shown and identify each type of x-ray production process being illustrated.

a) _____   b) _____

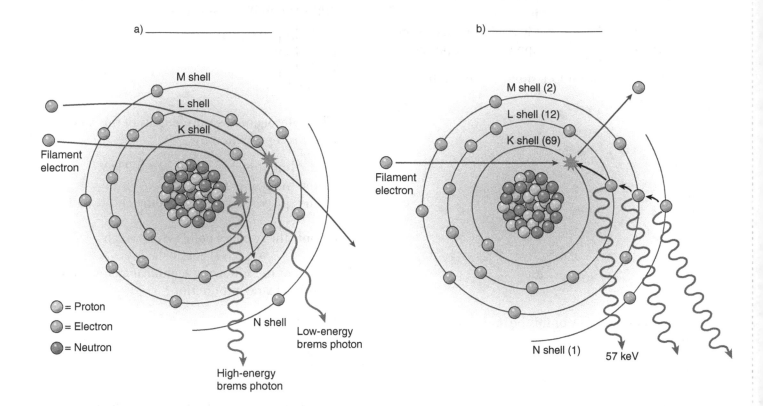

2. Complete the table by identifying the missing factors that influence the x-ray emission spectrum.

Factors Influencing the X-ray Emission Spectra	Effect(s) on the X-ray Emission Spectrum
1. _____	Controls the projectile electron energy, the intensity, the maximum energy, and the average energy of the x-ray beam.
2. _____	Controls the number of projectile electrons striking the anode and the intensity of the x-ray beam.
3. _____	Influences the intensity and average energy of the x-ray beam by filtering out low-energy photons.
4. _____	Influences the intensity and the average energy of the x-ray beam by making the x-ray tube more efficient.

3. Identify the technical factor change made in each of the x-ray emission spectra.

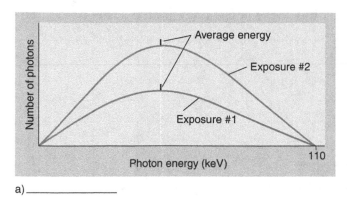

a) _____

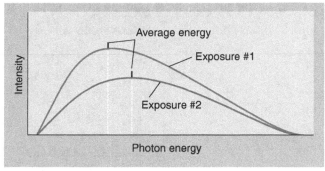

b) _____

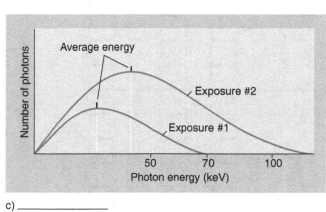

c) _____

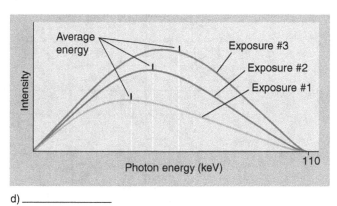

d) _____

Crossword Puzzle

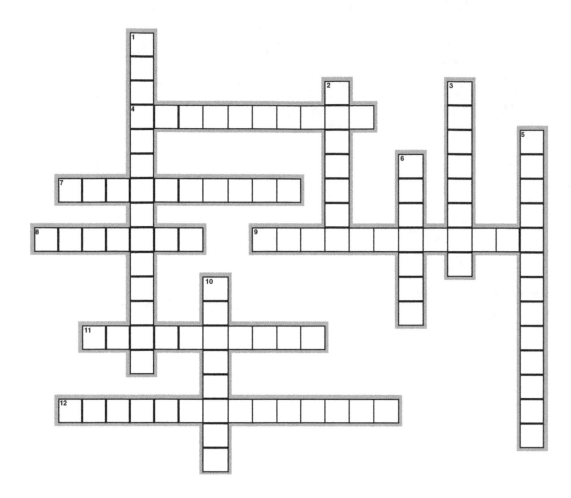

Across

4. Target material used in mammography
7. Eliminates low-energy photons by placing thin sheets of aluminum into the x-ray beam
8. Name for the process of an outer shell electron filling a vacancy left in an inner shell during a characteristic interaction
9. Graph which plots the number of x-ray photons produced as a function of their different energies
11. Brems radiation produces this type of spectrum
12. Type of radiation which results when an L-shell electron fills a K-shell vacancy

Down

1. Type of radiation which constitutes 90% of the x-rays produced
2. Describes the penetrability of the x-ray beam; controlled by the kVp setting
3. Describes the intensity of the x-ray beam; controlled by mAs
5. The kVp selected will be equal to this in keV; represents the maximum energy in the beam
6. Energy of motion; type of energy exhibited by incident electrons
10. Target material with a K-shell binding energy of 69.5 keV

PART III

Image Production

11

X-Ray Interactions with Matter

1. The interactions with matter of most importance in diagnostic radiology are:

   1. Compton
   2. Photoelectric
   3. Pair production

   a. 1, 2
   b. 1, 3
   c. 2, 3
   d. 1, 2, 3

2. The scatter photon produced as a result of a classical, or Thompson, interaction:

   a. has a shorter wavelength than the initial photon
   b. has a longer wavelength than the initial photon
   c. has the same wavelength as the initial photon
   d. goes on to create a characteristic photon

3. When an x-ray photon ejects an electron, the atom:

   a. becomes ionized
   b. becomes an unstable radioisotope
   c. transmutes to a new element
   d. emits additional electrons in response

4. What is (are) the product(s) of a photoelectric interaction?

   a. an electron
   b. an electron and a scattered x-ray
   c. a negative and positive
   d. a photoelectron and a characteristic x-ray

5. Which of the following results in total absorption of the primary x-ray photon?

   a. Compton scattering
   b. coherent scattering
   c. pair production
   d. photoelectric

6. _____ is more likely in the case of 40 keV x-rays incident on soft tissue.

   a. Coherent scattering
   b. Photoelectric interaction
   c. Compton scattering
   d. Characteristic radiation

7. Compton scattering:

   a. involves scattering from the atomic nucleus
   b. involves complete absorption of the incident x-ray
   c. involves a change in direction with no change in energy
   d. involves scattering from outer shell electrons

8. Recoil electrons are produced during:

   a. photoelectric interactions
   b. Compton scattering
   c. pair production
   d. coherent scattering

9. Annihilation radiation occurs when:

    a. an electron vacancy is filled in the K-shell by the L-shell
    b. the nucleus emits a particle
    c. a positron interacts with an electron
    d. two photons interact simultaneously with the same electron

10. The scatter photon produced as a result of a Compton interaction:

    a. has a shorter wavelength than the initial photon
    b. has a longer wavelength than the initial photon
    c. has the same wavelength as the initial photon
    d. goes on to create a characteristic photon

11. The x-ray interaction that involves no loss of energy or ionization is:

    a. coherent
    b. Compton
    c. photoelectric
    d. pair production

12. The pair production interaction has medical applications in which area of medical imaging of those listed below?

    a. magnetic resonance imaging
    b. computed tomography
    c. nuclear medicine
    d. sonography

13. What type of radiation is produced after a Compton interaction?

    a. bremsstrahlung
    b. characteristic
    c. primary
    d. secondary

14. How much initial energy is needed to initiate pair production?

    a. 0.51 MeV
    b. 1.02 MeV
    c. 2.01 MeV
    d. 10 MeV

15. Photoelectric effect occurs when:

    a. an x-ray photon causes an electron to vibrate
    b. an inner shell electron is ejected from its orbit
    c. a positive and negative electron are produced
    d. a nuclear fragment is emitted

16. Which of the following involves an ionization process?

    a. pair production
    b. classical scattering
    c. Compton scattering
    d. photodisintegration

17. The white or light gray areas on a radiograph are due primarily to:

    a. their similar densities
    b. photoelectric interactions
    c. Compton scattering
    d. image fog

18. The interaction that is Z# dependent is:

    a. coherent scattering
    b. Compton scattering
    c. photoelectric effect
    d. pair production annihilation

19. With increasing kVp and increasing photon energies:

    a. the proportion of Compton interactions increases compared to photoelectric interactions
    b. photoelectric interaction increase overall while Compton remains constant
    c. the proportion of Compton interactions decreases compared to an increase of photoelectric interactions
    d. as photoelectric interactions decrease, classical scattering becomes the predominant interaction

20. Classical scattering is more likely to occur:

    a. in bone and contrast materials
    b. at photon energies of 10 MeV and above
    c. in air-filled structures
    d. when photon energies are 10 keV or less

21. After the nucleus is excited during the photodisintegration process:

    a. a recoil electron is ejected
    b. gamma radiation is detected
    c. positive and negative electrons are produced
    d. a nuclear fragment is emitted

22. During a photoelectric interaction with a calcium atom, the photoelectron is found to have a KE of 15 keV. The binding energy of the K-shell is 4 keV. Based on this information, what was the energy of the initial photon?

    a. 11 keV
    b. 19 keV
    c. 60 keV
    d. 69 keV

23. An 85 keV incident photon interacts with an M-shell electron of potassium with a binding energy of 35 eV. The recoil electron exhibits a kinetic energy of 29 keV. What is the energy of the scatter photon?

    a. 21 keV
    b. 114 keV
    c. 56 keV
    d. 149 keV

24. Which substance's atoms are the most likely to undergo photoelectric interactions?

    a. barium
    b. soft tissue
    c. fat
    d. air

25. During a Compton interaction, the most energy will be given to the recoil electron when:

    a. the deflection angle is 0 degrees
    b. the deflection angle is at right angles to the object
    c. the deflection angle gets closer to 180 degrees
    d. a full 360 degrees is reached

26. An undesirable result of backscatter is:

    a. increased patient absorption
    b. increased recoil electron production
    c. increased characteristic photon production
    d. increased image fog

27. Technologist dose is the most likely to increase with the increased incidence of which type of interaction?

    a. pair production
    b. photoelectric
    c. Compton
    d. characteristic

28. Which part of the atom does the incident photon interact with when a pair production interaction is initiated?

    a. an outer shell's positive electron
    b. the nucleus
    c. an inner shell electron
    d. the nuclear field

29. The Compton interaction is characterized by:

    a. the absence of secondary radiation
    b. a positron-negatron pair
    c. partial energy transfer
    d. the Cascade effect

30. Thompson, or classical scatter, takes place when:

    a. an x-ray photon ionizes an electron
    b. a 1.02 MeV photon interacts with a nuclear field
    c. all of the incident photon's energy is transferred to the nucleus
    d. a low-energy photon interacts and rebounds with an orbital electron

Labeling

1. Label the lettered components for the classical scattering interaction shown.

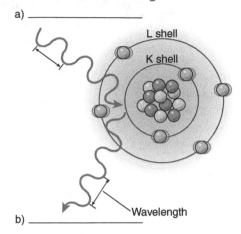

a) _____

b) _____

2. Identify the lettered components of the Compton interaction.

a) _____   b) _____

c) _____

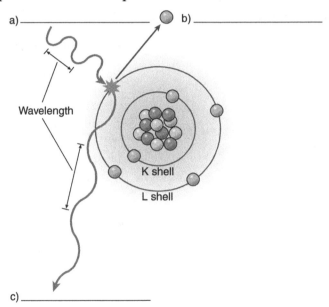

3. Label the steps in the process of the photoelectric interaction in the diagrams provided.

a) _____

b) _____

c) _____

d) _____

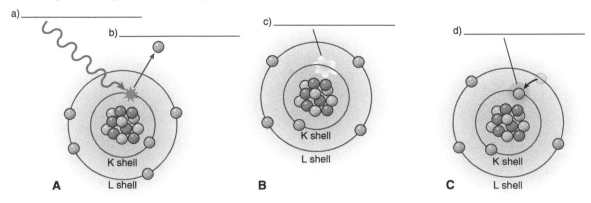

4. Complete the labels for the pair production interaction.

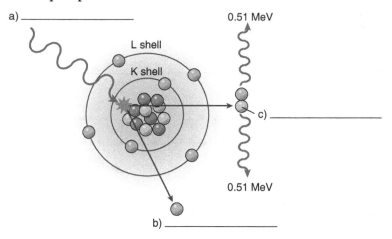

a) _____

0.51 MeV

L shell

K shell

c) _____

0.51 MeV

b) _____

5. Complete letters a and b representing the steps in a photodisintegration interaction.

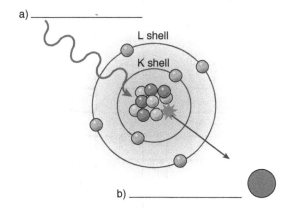

a) _____

L shell

K shell

b) _____

Crossword Puzzle

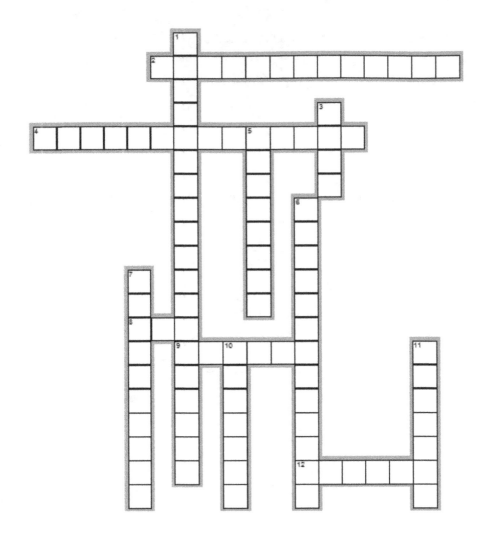

Across

2. Term used for the electron ejected during a photoelectric interaction
4. Interaction that results in a positive and negative electron
8. Results on a radiographic image that has been exposed to scatter or back scatter radiation
9. Another name for a Compton electron; a _____ electron
12. Contrast medium with a Z of 56

Down

1. Interaction that occurs in the nucleus of an atom
3. Type of tissue with the highest Z
5. Type of scatter where the scatter photon's wavelength is the same as the initial photon's wavelength
6. Interaction characterized by the total absorption of the incident photon
7. Describes the angle that determines the amount of energy that is transferred to the recoil electron during a Compton interaction
10. Occurs when a photon is only partially absorbed by tissue
11. The term used to describe the secondary radiation emitted by both the classical and Compton interactions

12

Beam Attenuation

1. _____ is the term used to describe the x-ray beam's reduction in intensity as it traverses through an object.

   a. Ionization
   b. Attenuation
   c. Elimination
   d. Transmission

2. Highly attenuating materials are called:

   a. radiopaque
   b. radiolucent
   c. radioactive
   d. radiosensitive

3. Transmission of radiation occurs when incident photons (are):

   a. completely absorbed by the nucleus
   b. partially absorbed by outer shell electrons
   c. deviated in their path by the nuclear field
   d. pass through the patient without interacting at all

4. Remnant radiation is made up of _____ radiation.

   1. Absorbed
   2. Scattered
   3. Transmitted

   a. 1, 2
   b. 1, 3
   c. 2, 3
   d. 1, 2, 3

5. The HVL is the amount of material required to reduce the:

   a. exit thickness to one-half the intensity
   b. exit intensity to one-half the thickness
   c. exit intensity to one-half the original intensity
   d. original intensity to one-half the exit intensity

6. The HVL in tissue is about:

   a. 1 cm
   b. 2 cm
   c. 3 cm
   d. 4 cm

7. What technical factor determines the penetrating ability of the x-ray beam?

   a. milliamperage
   b. time
   c. kilovoltage
   d. distance

8. Which of the following does not involve an attenuation process?

   a. transmission
   b. classical scattering
   c. Compton scattering
   d. photoelectric effect

9. The contrast between bone and soft tissue is due primarily to:

   a. their similar densities
   b. different abilities to absorb contrast materials
   c. the difference in their atomic numbers
   d. differences in part thickness

10. A radiolucent anatomical structure is one that:

   a. easily absorbs x-rays and prevents them from reaching the film
   b. easily transmits x-rays to the film
   c. interacts by the Compton effect
   d. filters out high-energy x-rays

11. Increasing kVp and increasing photon energies:

   a. increases Compton interactions and decreases subject contrast
   b. increases Compton interactions and increases subject contrast
   c. decreases Compton interactions and increases subject contrast
   d. decreases Compton interactions and decreases subject contrast

12. Which tissue is the most likely to attenuate the x-ray beam?

   a. bone
   b. soft tissue
   c. fat
   d. air

13. Differential absorption is most closely associated with which interaction with matter?

   a. pair production
   b. photoelectric
   c. Compton scattering
   d. classical scattering

14. Scatter radiation results in what change in the radiographic image?

   a. increased contrast
   b. increased fog
   c. increased brightness
   d. increased detail

15. The material/tissue with the lowest atomic number of those listed below is:

   a. air
   b. muscle
   c. lead
   d. fat

16. Total absorption of x-ray photons is more likely to occur in _____ structures.

   a. relatively dense
   b. air-filled
   c. water-based
   d. amorphous

17. The term for the radiation that exits the patient and interacts with the image receptor to form the radiographic image is:

   a. scatter
   b. remnant
   c. leakage
   d. primary

18. Contrast agents such as barium and iodine allow soft tissue and blood vessels to be visualized by:

   a. allowing more photons to be transmitted
   b. promoting more Compton interactions
   c. increasing the relative Z of the structures
   d. lowering the HVL's of the anatomy

19. Which of the following conditions will increase scatter radiation production?

   a. increased tissue Z#
   b. increased tissue density
   c. increased photon wavelength
   d. increased kVp

20. A photon exiting a patient is traveling in a new direction when it interacts with the image receptor. Based on this description, the photon can be described as:

   a. transmitted radiation
   b. leakage radiation
   c. scatter radiation
   d. nonionizing radiation

21. Approximately what percent of the primary beam passes through the patient without interacting at all?

    a. 99%
    b. 75%
    c. 25%
    d. 1%

22. If all of the x-ray photons were completely absorbed by the patient, the radiograph would appear:

    a. very dark and mostly black
    b. as a variety of gray shades
    c. very bright and mostly white
    d. blurred and mottled

23. Which of the following devices can be employed to remove scatter before it reaches the image receptor?

    a. filtration
    b. a grid
    c. collimator leaves
    d. a contrast agent

24. Based on the HVL absorption properties of tissue, when going from a 20 cm thickness to a 24 cm thickness, what change in technical factors would be needed to ensure adequate exposure is received by the image receptor?

    a. mAs would need to be doubled
    b. mAs would need to be halved
    c. kVp would need to be doubled
    d. kVp would need to be halved

25. The transmission of photons through a patient to the image receptor would be increased when:

    a. iodine is used as a contrast agent
    b. tissue density is increased
    c. tissue thickness is increased
    d. kVp is increased

Labeling

1. Label each type of remnant radiation illustrated in the diagram, indicating whether it is absorbed, scattered, or transmitted.

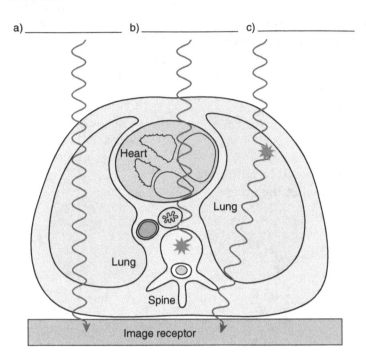

2. Starting with 1,000 incident photons, identify and label the number of photons remaining after each 4 cm of tissue attenuates the x-ray beam.

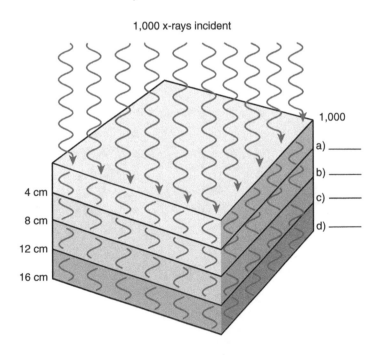

3. Complete the table, indicating each factor's effect on beam attenuation

Factor	Beam Attenuation	Absorption	Transmission
Tissue Thickness			
Increasing thickness	_____	_____	_____
Decreasing thickness	_____	_____	_____
Tissue Type (Z number)			
Increasing Z number	_____	_____	_____
Decreasing Z number	_____	_____	_____
Tissue Density			
Increasing density	_____	_____	_____
Decreasing density	_____	_____	_____
X-ray Photon Energy			
Increasing energy	_____	_____	_____
Decreasing energy	_____	_____	_____

Crossword Puzzle

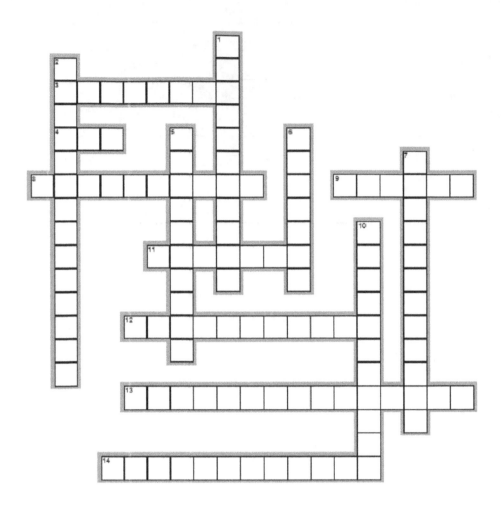

Across

3. Occurs when a photon's energy is completely transferred to the tissue and no longer exists
4. Unwanted density deposited on the image; more likely to occur when kVp is increased
8. Term used to describe structures that absorb photons
9. Contrast agent that is radiopaque
11. Secondary radiation that exits the patient
12. The ability of x-rays to go through matter; kVp increases or decreases this quality
13. The ability to distinguish structures as a result of the absorption characteristics
14. Occurs when radiation passes through a patient without interacting at all

Down

1. Quality used to describe materials with low attenuation properties
2. Amount of material required to reduce the x-ray beam intensity to one-half its original intensity
5. Occurs when a photon is only partially absorbed by tissue
6. Tissue quality that is measured in grams per cubic centimeter (g/cc)
7. _____ absorption is a process that compares the x-ray photons that interact photoelectrically to those that do not
10. The gradual absorption of photons as they pass through matter

13

Radiographic Image Characteristics

1. Optical density:

   a. is always lowest at the shoulder of a characteristic curve
   b. is the logarithm of the ratio of incident to transmitted light
   c. can be measured with a sensitometer
   d. is not affected by light or radiation fog

2. The optical density of a film is measured with a:

   a. sensitometer
   b. densitometer
   c. penetrometer
   d. photometer

3. A radiograph having a density of 1.0 will transmit what percentage of illuminator light?

   a. 1%
   b. 10%
   c. 100%
   d. 1,000%

4. A characteristic curve of a film relates:

   a. optical density to the light transmitted through the film
   b. subject contrast to tissue density
   c. optical density to developer temperature
   d. optical density to log relative exposure

5. The diagnostic range of exposures on the straight-line portion of the sensitometric curve falls between:

   a. 0.2 and 3.0
   b. 0.25 and 2.5
   c. 1.0 and 3.0
   d. 2.5 and 5.0

6. Radiographic contrast consists of a combination of:

   a. subject contrast and scattering
   b. subject contrast and film contrast
   c. film contrast and grid contrast
   d. density and mAs

7. Subject contrast depends on:

   a. tissue thickness
   b. tissue density
   c. tissue atomic number
   d. all of the above

8. Long-scale contrast radiographs are obtained using:

   a. increased mAs
   b. decreased mAs
   c. increased kVp
   d. decreased kVp

9. The straight-line portion of the characteristic curve of a film can be used to:

   a. determine its base + fog measurement
   b. measure its contrast
   c. find its maximum density
   d. determine sharpness

10. The contrast of a film:

    a. is measured by evaluating the slope of the straight-line portion on the characteristic curve
    b. is always identical to its speed
    c. is directly proportional to its latitude
    d. describes the image's blackness

11. A high-contrast film has a _____ latitude.

    a. wide
    b. narrow
    c. long
    d. low

12. A characteristic curve optical density measurement of 0.3 would most likely be found at the:

    a. toe
    b. straight-line portion
    c. shoulder
    d. D_{max}

13. The shoulder of the characteristic curve represents:

    a. a film's base + fog measurement
    b. the area of highest film resolution
    c. a film's latitude of exposure
    d. the maximum densities achievable

14. The device that is used to consistently produce a series of density steps progressing from clear to black best describes the:

    a. densitometer
    b. thermometer
    c. sensitometer
    d. optimeter

15. A radiograph has been determined to have high contrast. This means that the density differences between structures are:

    a. relatively small
    b. exactly equal
    c. large
    d. greater than 0.5 on a densitometer reading

16. In general, as screen speed increases, density _____.

    a. decreases
    b. increases
    c. remains constant

17. A variation from the true shape of the part being radiographed is defined as:

    a. misrepresentation
    b. facsimile
    c. magnification
    d. distortion

18. If the central ray is not placed so that it is directed through the center of the anatomy, the radiographic quality most affected will be:

    a. density
    b. contrast
    c. detail
    d. distortion

19. An increase in the source-to-image/receptor distance will:

    a. increase penumbra
    b. increase blur
    c. decrease penumbra
    d. no change in penumbra

20. Which of the following would have the most effect on magnification of the image on a finished radiograph?

    a. object image-receptor distance
    b. motion
    c. focal spot size
    d. system speed

21. To calculate the magnification factor:

    a. divide the SID by the OID
    b. divide the object size by the image size
    c. divide the SID by the SOD
    d. divide the OID by the SID

22. A radiograph of the sella turcica was performed using an SID of 40 in. The sella turcica has a 10 in OID. What is the magnification factor of the sella turcica?

    a. 0.25
    b. 0.75
    c. 1.33
    d. 4.0

23. Which of the following has/have no effect on sharpness of detail?

    a. penumbra
    b. motion
    c. density
    d. lp/mm

24. Size distortion will be affected by all EXCEPT the following:

    a. SID
    b. SOD
    c. OID
    d. FSS

25. A UGI image is blurred. Based on the type of exam being conducted, to increase sharpness of detail the technologist could:

    a. decrease exposure time
    b. use a single screen cassette
    c. decrease kVp and mAs
    d. decrease SID

26. Which of the following combinations of factors will provide the greatest detail?

    a. short SID, short OID, small FSS
    b. long SID, short OID, small FSS
    c. long SID, long OID, large FSS
    d. short SID, long OID, large FSS

For Questions 27 through 30, indicate whether the property is described by and/or can be evaluated by the characteristic curve. Answer A for true or B for false.

27. _____ Focal spot size

28. _____ Contrast

29. _____ Base plus fog level

30. _____ Speed

Labeling

1. Label the parts of the characteristic curve:

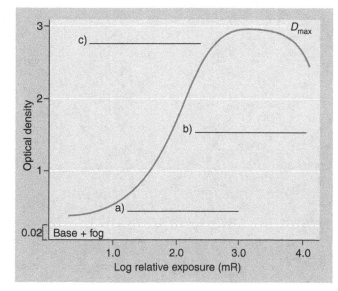

2. Identify the type of distance indicated in the diagram.

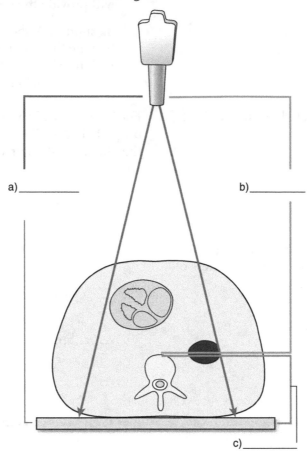

a) _____   b) _____

c) _____

3. **Indicate whether the Focal spot or SID and OID is large or small based on the diagrams.**

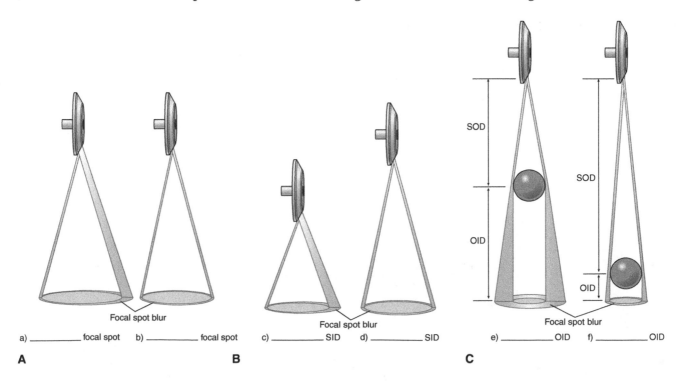

a) _____ focal spot   b) _____ focal spot   c) _____ SID   d) _____ SID   e) _____ OID   f) _____ OID

A   **B**   **C**

4. Identify whether the anatomy is elongated or foreshortened.

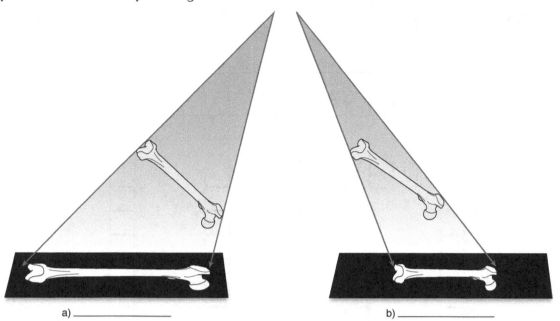

a) _____   b) _____

5. Complete the table indicating whether the factor will increase or decrease the image qualities shown or if they will remain unchanged.

Factor	Patient Dose	Magnification	Film Density
Film speed	_____	_____	_____
Patient thickness	_____	_____	_____
Focal spot size	_____	_____	_____
SID			
OID			
mAs			
Exposure time			
kVp			

Crossword Puzzle

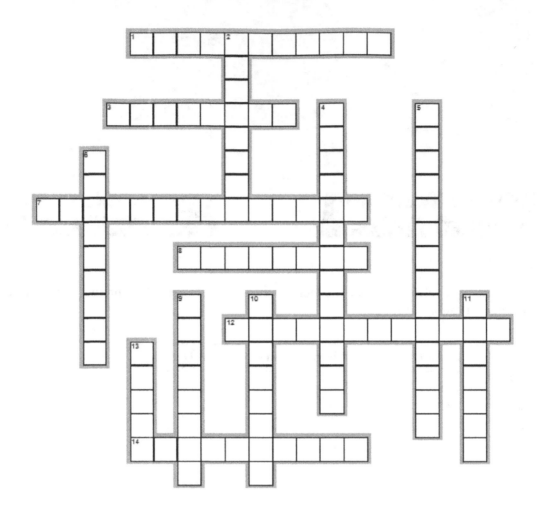

Across

1. A form of involuntary motion
3. The range of exposures that produce an acceptable radiograph
7. _____ curve; plots the relative log exposure on the *x*-axis and the optical density of the film on the *y*-axis
8. Tube angle toward the head
12. Aluminum step wedge
14. Misrepresentation of an object on an image, either in its size or in its shape

Down

2. Portion of the sensitometric curve where D_{max} is measured
4. Type of distortion that makes an object appear larger than its actual size
5. Type of shape distortion that makes an object appear smaller than its actual size in one axis
6. Measured using lp/mm
9. Density differences on an image
10. Blur; occurs around the edge of an image
11. Degree of blackness on an image
13. Value used to measure film's sensitivity to exposure

14

Image Exposure

1. The primary factor that controls density is:

   a. kVp
   b. mAs
   c. grids
   d. SID

2. The primary factory that controls image contrast is:

   a. kVp
   b. mAs
   c. SID
   d. focal spot size

3. In order to increase contrast, the technologist should:

   a. increase mAs
   b. decrease kVp
   c. increase SID
   d. decrease grid ratio

In Questions 4 through 6, match the technical changes with the effect it controls and produces on the image.

4. _____ Increased mAs

5. _____ Increased kVp

6. _____ Decreased kVp

   a. Increased density
   b. Less contrast, longer scale of contrast
   c. Decreased density
   d. Shorter contrast scale, greater contrast

7. Which of the following occurs when a technologist increases the technique from 200 to 400 mA?

   a. the x-ray photons become more penetrating and increase density
   b. fewer photons reach the image receptor because kVp is automatically decreased by the x-ray circuit
   c. more x-ray photons are produced that increases density
   d. lower energy photons are filtered out, making the beam more energetic

8. What mA station is set if the total mAs is 75 mAs and the time is 250 ms?

   a. 18.7
   b. 100
   c. 300
   d. 1,000

9. To alter the technical factors so that a breathing technique can be set, the technologist should:

   a. increase time and decrease mA
   b. increase mA and decrease time
   c. increase mAs and decrease kVp
   d. increase kVp and decrease mAs

10. What combination of exposure factors will produce the highest density and/or exposure to the image receptor?

    a. 200 mA, 250 ms
    b. 300 mA, 120 ms
    c. 150 mA, 300 ms
    d. 100 mA, 450 ms

11. The minimum percent change in mAs required to see a noticeable change in film density is about:

    a. 50%
    b. 30%
    c. 0%
    d. 20%

12. If the original technique used was 60 kVp at 25 mAs, which new technique will result in a film density two times darker?

    a. 64 kVp at 25 mAs
    b. 60 kVp at 50 mAs
    c. 60 kVp at 33 mAs
    d. 60 kVp at 75 mAs

13. If the original technique is 65 kVp, 200 mA, and 175 ms, and the technologist wishes to double density or the exposure to the IR using kVp ONLY, the new technique would be:

    a. 65 kVp, 200 mA, and 350 ms
    b. 75 kVp, 100 mA, and 350 ms
    c. 75 kVp, 200 mA, and 175 ms
    d. 85 kVp, 200 mA, and 88 ms

14. When kVp is increased and all other factors are unchanged:

    a. density increases and contrast increases
    b. density increases and contrast decreases
    c. density decreases and contrast increases
    d. density decreases and contrast decreases

15. In order to maintain density, when one increases kVp from 70 to 80 kVp, one must:

    a. increase mAs by two times
    b. decrease mAs to 1/4 the original
    c. increase mAs by four times
    d. decrease mAs to 1/2 the original

16. An exposure of 85 kVp and 200 mAs produces a correct density but too much contrast. What mAs should be used if the kVp is raised to 100 kVp?

    a. 50
    b. 100
    c. 200
    d. 400

17. If the distance from the source is increased by a factor of 2, the mAs must be _____ to maintain the same density

    a. increased by a factor of 2
    b. decreased by a factor of 2
    c. increased by a factor of 4
    d. decreased by a factor of 4

18. If the distance from the source is decreased by a factor of 2, the mAs must be _____ to maintain the same image density

    a. increased by a factor of 2
    b. decreased by a factor of 2
    c. increased by a factor of 4
    d. decreased by a factor of 4

19. If the SID is increased from 40″ to 60″ and the original mAs used is 20 mAs, what new mAs is needed to maintain density?

    a. 10 mAs
    b. 26 mAs
    c. 40 mAs
    d. 80 mAs

20. Which of the following techniques would produce the same density as 500 mA at 0.03 s?

    a. 300 mA at 0.05 s
    b. 100 mA at 0.015 s
    c. 200 mA at 0.10 s
    d. 250 mA at 0.6 s

21. The greater the number of photons (intensity) that reach the image receptor, the:

    a. greater image penumbra
    b. greater the contrast
    c. greater the density
    d. lower the contrast

22. The factor that alters x-ray beam penetration is

    a. mAs
    b. kVp
    c. distance
    d. focal spot size

23. An exposure of 40″ SID 200 mA 2s 80 kVp is changed to 40″ SID 100 mA 2s. What kVp should be chosen to produce the same image?

    a. 70 kVp
    b. 80 kVp
    c. 92 kVp
    d. 100 kVp

24. At 60″, the x-ray intensity is 90 mR. What is the intensity at 36″?

    a. 36 mR
    b. 18 mR
    c. 250 mR
    d. 360 mR

25. If insufficient photons reach the image receptor, what form of image noise becomes apparent?

    a. radiographic fog
    b. Compton scatter
    c. excessive density
    d. quantum mottle

26. You are completing a T-spine examination and have always had great success using a breathing technique for the lateral. However, the new hospital where you are at has only a suspended technique posted:

    200 mA   70 kVp   0.25 s.
    If the lowest mA station available is 25 mA, what will your new technique be to allow a breathing exposure to be taken?

    a. 25 mA, 70 kVp, 2.0 s
    b. 25 mA, 90 kVp, 0.25 s
    c. 25 mA, 70 kVp, 0.002 s
    d. 25 mA, 60 kVp, 3.0 s

27. The digital imaging function that corrects an overexposed or underexposed radiograph so that density and image brightness appear optimal is:

    a. the filament circuit's resistor
    b. its dynamic range
    c. automatic rescaling
    d. straight-line portion adaptation

28. kVp selection in digital imaging systems:

    a. affects contrast in the same manner as film/screen systems
    b. has less impact on image appearance due to digital's wide dynamic range
    c. is more variable due to the use of post-processing software
    d. has more effect on beam quantity than beam quality

29. Which of the following technique changes would reduce patient dose and be supported by the use of digital imaging without changing overall image quality?

    a. increasing all kVp selections by 15% while reducing mAs to one-half
    b. increasing all 40″ SID's to 48″ and applying the Direct Square Law
    c. doubling all mAs values while reducing kVp by 15%
    d. increasing mAs by 30% to 50% and applying post-processing software

30. The preferred technical factor change used to eliminate quantum mottle in a film/screen or digital image would be to:

    a. increase kVp by 15% while leaving mAs constant
    b. decrease SID by 50% and applying the Direct Square Law
    c. use two times the exposure time but one-half of the mA
    d. increase mAs but leave kVp constant

Labeling

1. Evaluate the foot radiographs. Based on their densities, label each foot image with its probable mA values given the following values: 12, 6, and 3 mAs

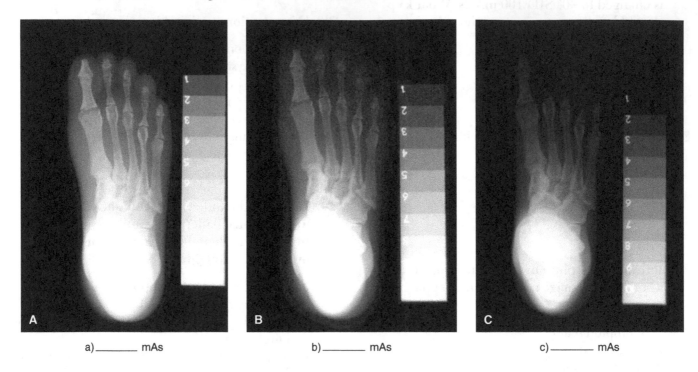

a) _____ mAs   b) _____ mAs   c) _____ mAs

2. Evaluate the knee radiographs. Based on their densities, label each knee image with its probable kVp values given the following values: 65, 75, and 55 kVp.

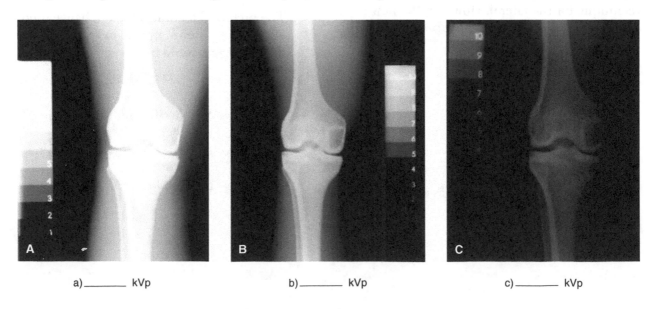

a) _____ kVp   b) _____ kVp   c) _____ kVp

3. Complete the table indicating whether the factor will increase or decrease the image qualities shown or if they will remain unchanged.

Factor	Density Change	Contrast Change
mA increase	_____	_____
mA decrease	_____	_____
Time increase	_____	_____
Time decrease	_____	_____
kVp increase	_____	_____
kVp decrease	_____	_____
SID increase	_____	_____
SID decrease	_____	_____
Focal spot increase	_____	_____
Focal spot decrease	_____	_____

Crossword Puzzle

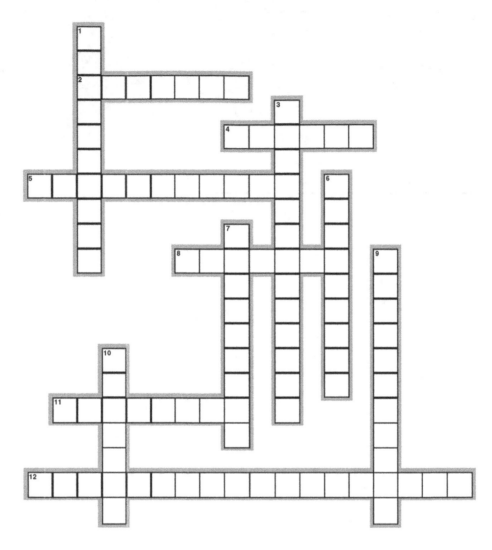

Across

2. The relationship between mA and time when total mAs and density are maintained
4. This law allows density or exposure to the IR to be maintained when SID changes; Direct _____ Law
5. Term used to describe the x-ray beam's ability to pass through structures
8. This quality of digital imaging systems is a reason that kVp no longer controls contrast to the same degree; wide _____ range
11. The controlling factor for this radiographic image quality is kVp
12. This rule is applied to kVp when density must be increased by a factor of two (three words)

Down

1. Opposite of density; typically used to describe the darkness or lightness of digital images
3. Form of radiographic noise; causes images to appear grainy (two words)
6. The computer software accomplishes this in digital imaging, making an over- or underexposed image appears acceptable: automatic _____
7. Term used to describe the number of or quantity of photons in the x-ray beam
9. The full name for mA
10. mAs is the controlling technical factor of this radiographic image quality

Controlling Scatter Radiation

15

1. Increasing the field size will _____ the amount of scatter.

   a. increase
   b. decrease
   c. unchanged

2. Increasing the x-ray beam energy will _____ the amount of scatter.

   a. increase
   b. decrease
   c. unchanged

3. A decrease in patient thickness will _____ the amount of scatter.

   a. increase
   b. decrease
   c. unchanged

4. Most of the scattered radiation reaching the image receptor during an x-ray exposure has an energy:

   a. greater than the primary beam
   b. equal to that of the primary beam
   c. less than that of the primary beam
   d. equal to 1.02 MeV or above

5. The most common field size limitation device in use is the:

   a. light-localizing variable aperture collimator
   b. aperture diaphragm
   c. Potter-Bucky diaphragm
   d. a flared-flange extension cone

6. The grid ratio is the ratio of the:

   a. height of the lead strips to the distance between the lead strips
   b. height of the lead strips to the width of the lead strips
   c. height of the plastic strips to the width of the plastic strips
   d. thickness of the grid to the width of the cassette

7. A grid should usually be employed in which of the following circumstances?

   1. When radiographing a large or dense body part
   2. When using high kVp
   3. When less patient dose is required

   a. 1 and 2 only
   b. 2 and 3 only
   c. 3 only
   d. 1, 2, and 3

8. The undesirable reduction of density on one or both sides of a radiograph due to misalignment of the x-ray beam to a grid is called:

   a. primary beam scatter
   b. grid cutoff
   c. grid frequency
   d. grid fog

9. Grid cutoff can result from:

   a. a focused grid used at the wrong SID
   b. using small SIDs with a parallel grid
   c. an upside-down focused grid
   d. all of the above

10. A grid is designed with lead strips 0.5 mm apart. The height of the lead strips is 8 mm. What is the grid ratio?

    a. 16:1
    b. 8:1
    c. 12:1
    d. 10:1

11. When a grid with a higher grid ratio is used, the radiation dose to the patient will _____ and the radiographic contrast will _____

    a. increase; decrease
    b. increase; increase
    c. decrease; increase
    d. decrease; decrease

12. When an 8:1 grid ratio is replaced with a 16:1 grid

    a. the mAs must be increased
    b. the mAs must be decreased
    c. the radiographic contrast is unchanged
    d. none of the above

13. The use of grids has no effect on:

    a. image contrast
    b. scatter radiation clean-up
    c. x-ray beam energy
    d. image gray scale

A radiographic examination using a focused grid produces images with densities that are lighter toward the edges. Questions 14 through 18 list various factors as possible causes. Answer A for true if the factor could cause this appearance and B for false if it does not.

14. _____ Patient motion

15. _____ Incorrect SID

16. _____ SID in focusing range

17. _____ Grid placed upside down

18. _____ Increased focal spot size

19. Which of the following are used to improve contrast and reduce scatter?

    a. collimation and filtration
    b. grids and collimation
    c. filtration and grids
    d. high kVp and long SID

20. A grid that is constructed so that all of the grid strips match the divergence of the x-ray beam would be a/an:

    a. focused grid
    b. linear grid
    c. oscillating grid
    d. crossed grid

21. Which of the following will cause an increase in image contrast?

    a. increased scatter
    b. smaller grid ratios
    c. increased grid cutoff
    d. smaller field sizes

22. An exposure made at 70 kVp and 10 mAs without a grid produces an acceptable density, but with too much scatter. A second exposure using a 12:1 grid is used. What should the new mAs be to maintain density?

    a. 2 mAs
    b. 25 mAs
    c. 50 mAs
    d. 100 mAs

23. A technique of 400 mA and 100 ms is used with a 16:1 grid, if an exam is done using a 6:1 grid, what new mAs is needed to maintain density?

    a. 2 mAs
    b. 20 mAs
    c. 0.2 mAs
    d. 200 mAs

24. The number of grid strips or grid lines per inch or centimeter is called:

    a. grid ratio
    b. grid frequency
    c. line pair
    d. line focus principle

25. A focused grid:

    a. is always used with thin body parts
    b. must be used with the correct SID
    c. requires a decrease in mAs compared to the no-grid mAs
    d. has a bucky factor of zero

26. The bucky factor:

    a. indicates how much contrast will increase when comparing nongrid and grid exposures
    b. indicates how fast the grid is moving
    c. indicates how much mAs must be increased compared to nongrid techniques
    d. indicates how much scatter radiation is present

27. A 12:1 ratio grid is substituted for an 8:1 grid. If identical technical factors are used, the new film will possess a higher:

    a. radiographic contrast
    b. radiographic density
    c. percentage of scatter
    d. all of the above

28. Which of the following is a disadvantage of using a moving grid?

    a. increased detail
    b. decreased SID
    c. increased OID
    d. increased grid cutoff

29. The wall bucky in your department is supplied with a 12:1 grid with a specified focal range of 65 to 80 inches. You perform an emergency upright shoulder examination at an appropriate technique. Which of the following statements would correctly describe the appearance of the finished radiograph?

    a. grid cutoff on one side of the image
    b. grid cutoff on all four sides of the image
    c. grid cutoff along both edges of the film
    d. density will be maintained throughout the image (i.e., no change)

30. The air gap technique is utilized to reduce scatter:

    a. with the use of a grid
    b. without the use of a grid
    c. with a short SID
    d. with air filtering out the scatter

Labeling

1. Label the lettered components of the diagram illustrating the relationship of the patient, the image receptor, and grid materials.

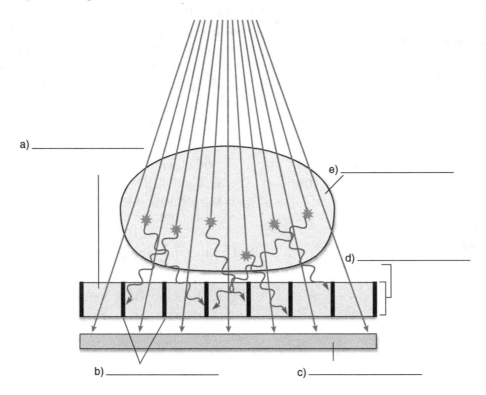

a) _____

e) _____

d) _____

b) _____   c) _____

2. Label letters a through d, indicating whether the dimension shown is "height" or "distance."

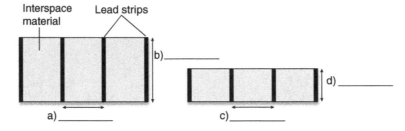

Interspace material   Lead strips

b) _____

a) _____

d) _____

c) _____

3. Complete the table by listing the appropriate bucky factor (grid conversion factor) by each grid shown.

Grid Ratio	Bucky Factor or GCF
None	_____
5:1	_____
6:1	_____
8:1	_____
12:1	_____
16:1	_____

4. Describe the radiographic density that would be observed if the grid error causes listed in the second column occurred during a radiographic examination.

Optical Density	Possible Causes
_____	Parallel grid at too short SID
_____	Upside-down focused grid
_____	Focused grid outside focal distance range
_____	Grid center not aligned with central axis
_____	Grid not perpendicular to central axis

Crossword Puzzle

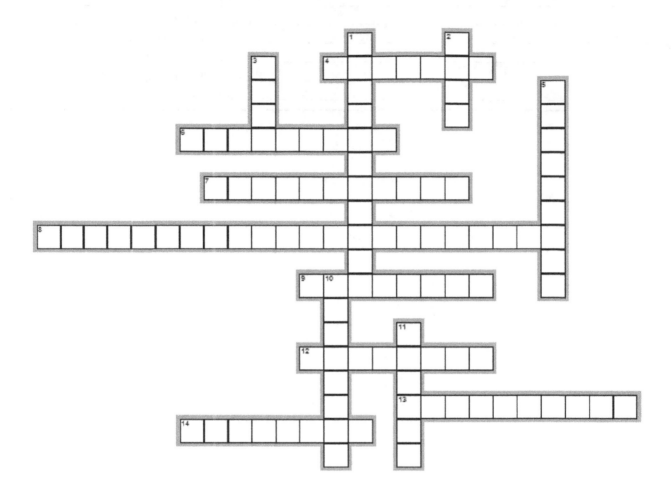

Across

4. Type of grid that must be used at a specific SID
6. Calculated using the formula: h/D
7. Circular bucky motion
8. Device that automatically collimates to the size of the image receptor placed in the bucky grid
9. Image quality which is the most improved when a grid is used
12. Interspace material commonly used in grid construction
13. General term for a grid error that causes a loss of density on one or both sides of an image
14. Type of grid where the lead strips are laid down in a line

Down

1. Defines the size and shape of the primary beam; used to limit field size
2. Radiopaque material used to construct a grid
3. Device made of lead strips to absorb scatter radiation
5. Number of lead strips per centimeter
10. Type of grid error that occurs when the grid is not perpendicular to the central ray
11. A scatter reduction technique that utilizes a large OID

Radiographic Film and Processing

16

1. **Film base:**

   a. provides support for the film emulsion
   b. must have a high opacity
   c. is constituted of gelatin
   d. is chemically reactive

2. **The most common halide used in radiographic film emulsions is/are:**

   a. rare earth crystals
   b. gelatin
   c. silver bromide
   d. calcium tungstate

3. **The sensitivity speck is a sensitive region:**

   a. in the polyester film base
   b. in the film cassette
   c. on the silver halide crystal
   d. in the developer solution

4. **The latent image is the distribution of:**

   a. exposed and unexposed crystals in the undeveloped film
   b. blackened silver halide crystals after development
   c. blackened silver halide crystals in the developer solution
   d. blackened and unexposed silver halide crystals on the undeveloped x-ray film

5. **A high-speed film is one which:**

   a. requires a high kVp to produce a given exposure
   b. requires a very short development time
   c. requires a relatively low exposure to produce a given density
   d. requires a relatively high exposure to produce a given density

6. **Spectral matching of the film and screens refer to matching of the:**

   a. film crystal size to the phosphor crystal size
   b. emulsion thickness to the phosphor thickness
   c. color of the cassette to the film sensitivity
   d. film sensitivity to the color of the light emitted by the phosphor

7. **A 600-speed system is in general use in your department, but on a particular exam, you switch to a 200-speed system. To maintain density, you will have to:**

   a. increase technique by 3 times
   b. increase technique by 1/3
   c. increase technique by 400 times
   d. decrease technique by 1/3

8. Your current technique of 1.5 mAs at 56 kVp is used for a hand utilizing a system speed of 400. A suspicious area on a hand requires a better film so you switch to a system with a speed of 150. What new technique is required to maintain original density?

   a. 0.6 mAs
   b. 6.0 mAs
   c. 4.0 mAs
   d. 40 mAs

9. Which of the following would enhance resolution the MOST?

   a. use a film with larger silver halide crystals
   b. use slower-speed film
   c. use a film with a thicker emulsion
   d. use a safelight filter

10. The purpose of processing and development is to:

   a. create the latent image
   b. enhance radiographic base + fog
   c. minimize artifact formation
   d. make the latent image visible

11. Which of the following films/screen combinations would require the highest mAs in order to achieve the proper exposure?

   a. detail
   b. medium speed
   c. high speed

12. Scratches on the screen will appear as _____ artifacts.

   a. negative density
   b. positive density
   c. quantum mottle
   d. fog density

13. Which of the following is not related to the construction of an intensifying screen?

   a. plastic base
   b. phosphor layer
   c. emulsion layer
   d. reflective layer

14. The reflective layer utilizes which of the following materials?

   1. Magnesium oxide
   2. Calcium tungstate
   3. Titanium dioxide

   a. 1, 2
   b. 2, 3
   c. 1, 3
   d. 1, 2, 3

15. The purpose of a lead foil liner in the back of a film cassette is to:

   a. absorb backscatter radiation
   b. protect the patient
   c. promote photoelectric interactions
   d. reflect light photons back onto the film

16. Which of the following characteristics is desired in screen phosphor materials?

   1. High atomic number
   2. Longer phosphorescence times
   3. High conversion efficiencies

   a. 1, 2
   b. 1, 3
   c. 2, 3
   d. 1, 2, 3

17. In general, as screen speed increases, density _____ and detail _____.

   a. decreases, decreases
   b. decreases, increases
   c. increases, increases
   d. increases, decreases

18. The primary reason intensifying screens are used is to:

   a. reduce patient dose
   b. increase spatial resolution
   c. allow higher mAs techniques
   d. convert light to x-rays

19. Convert the following technique used on a 500-speed imaging system to a 150-speed imaging system so that density is maintained: 60 kVp 9 mAs

   a. 60 kVp 4.5 mAs
   b. 60 kVp 18 mAs
   c. 60 kVp 30 mAs
   d. 70 kVp 45 mAs

20. Which of the following is the most likely to result in quantum mottle?

    a. a damaged protective coat
    b. poor film-screen contact
    c. large phosphor crystals
    d. low mAs values

21. The substance with the highest conversion efficiency is the most likely to be:

    a. calcium tungstate
    b. lanthanum
    c. lead
    d. magnesium oxide

22. The most appropriate measure for an intensifying screen's spatial resolution is (its):

    a. conversion efficiency
    b. speed
    c. lp/mm
    d. light photon energy

23. If there is light leak in a cassette, this would be detected due to:

    a. increased image fog
    b. decreased detail or spatial resolution
    c. white, negative density artifacts
    d. mesh-like artifacts

24. A film cassette must have which of the following qualities?

    1. A radiolucent front
    2. Light-proof
    3. Even pressure across the film

    a. 1, 2
    b. 1, 3
    c. 2, 3
    d. 1, 2, 3

25. Solution replenishment occurs in an automatic processor that is controlled by the activation of a:

    a. master roller
    b microswitch
    c. circulation pump
    d. guideshoe

26. Total processing time is controlled by which automatic processor system?

    a. thermostat
    b. transport
    c. recirculation
    d. replenishment

27. To meet EPA guidelines, a silver recovery unit is required to be connected to the:

    a. developer
    b. fixer
    c. water
    d. dryer

28. If a darkroom safelight emitted too much light, what undesirable effect occurs?

    a. radiographic fog
    b. inadequate density
    c. quantum mottle
    d. photoelectric

29. A common source of artifacts in an automatic processor is/are the:

    a. microswitch
    b. laser light
    c. guideshoes
    d. GBX filter

30. The developer temperature in most 90-second automatic processors is in the range of:

    a. 68°F to 72°F (23°C to 25°C)
    b. 80°F (28°C +/− 5°C)
    c. 92°F to 95°F (28°C +/− 5°C)
    d. 110°F to 120°F (43°C to 50°C)

Labeling

1. Label each layer of the double-emulsion film shown:

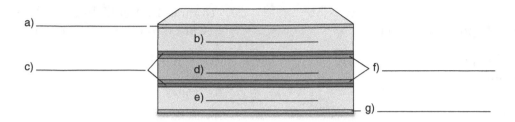

a) _____

b) _____

c) _____

d) _____

e) _____

f) _____

g) _____

2. Complete the table demonstrating the relationships of crystal size and emulsion to film speed and resolution

	Crystal Size		Emulsion Layer	
	Small	Large	Thin	Thick
Speed	____	____	____	____
Resolution	____	____	____	____

3. Identify the lettered components of an intensifying screen.

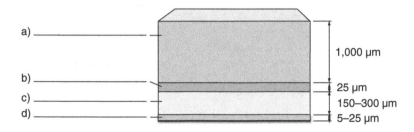

a) _____

b) _____

c) _____

d) _____

1,000 μm

25 μm

150–300 μm

5–25 μm

4. Label the processor components:

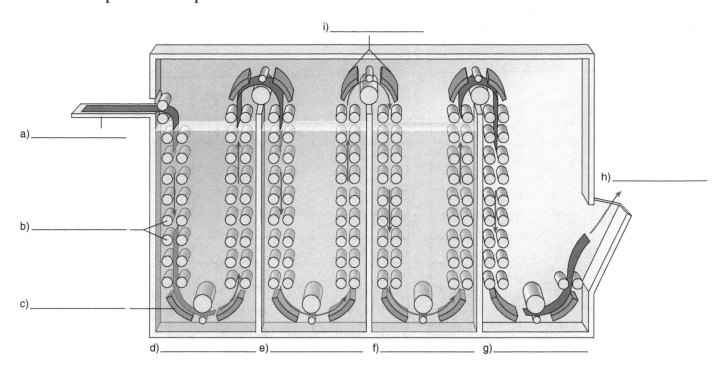

Crossword Puzzle

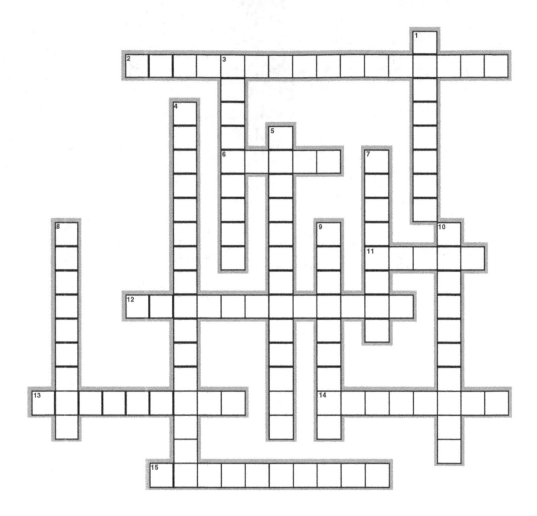

Across

2. Principle that film should be sensitive to the wavelengths of light emitted by the intensifying screen (two words)
6. Numerical measure used to describe film/screen sensitivity to exposure
11. Processing solution responsible for clearing unexposed silver halide crystals
12. Production of light due to the stimulation of a crystal by x-rays
13. Material used for the base of radiographic film and intensifying screen phosphors
14. Made of silver halide crystals suspended in gelatin
15. Component of an intensifying screen; redirects the light back to the film: _____ layer

Down

1. Crystal that converts x-rays to light
3. Processing system that controls time that the film is in each solution
4. Blue light–emitting phosphor developed by Thomas Edison (two words)
5. Processing system responsible for ensuring fresh chemistry is regularly added to the developer and fixer
7. Any unwanted information or density(ies) on a radiograph
8. Metal component responsible for causing scratches on film during automatic processing if it becomes misaligned
9. Processing solution for making the latent image visible
10. Measured using lp/mm: spatial _____

Radiographic Technique

17

1. Which of the following is NOT a subject factor that affects radiographic quality?

   a. patient thickness
   b. patient height
   c. body habitus
   d. patient age

2. In an asthenic patient,

   a. an excess of fatty and adipose tissue is present
   b. all tissue absorption factors would be normal
   c. caliper measurements would be higher than normal
   d. decreased technique settings would be appropriate

3. The patient body habitus indicative of an increased patient thickness is:

   a. hypersthenic
   b. sthenic
   c. hyposthenic
   d. asthenic

4. Which of the following most accurately describes the relationship between part thickness and x-ray beam attenuation?

   a. increased part thickness causes increased attenuation
   b. decreased part thickness causes increased attenuation
   c. increased part thickness causes decreased attenuation

5. Which of the following contribute to the radiographic (subject) contrast present on a radiograph?

   1. Atomic number of tissues radiographed
   2. Any pathologic processes
   3. Degree of muscle development

   a. 1 and 2
   b. 1 and 3
   c. 2 and 3
   d. 1, 2, and 3

6. For which pathology(ies) below would a decrease in technique probably be required to obtain desired density levels?

   1. Osteoporosis
   2. Emphysema
   3. Osteopetrosis
   4. Ascites

   a. 1 and 2 only
   b. 3 and 4 only
   c. 2 and 4 only
   d. 1, 2, and 3

7. To alter the technical factors so that a pediatric technique can be set, the technologist should:

   a. decrease kVp and increase mAs
   b. decrease mAs and decrease kVp
   c. increase mAs and increase kVp
   d. increase kVp and decrease mAs

101

8. All of the following are methods to reduce motion during a pediatric examination EXCEPT:

   a. using Pig-o-stats
   b. using longer exposure times
   c. using detent functions
   d. using clear instructions

9. The minimum percent change in mAs required to see a noticeable change in film density is about:

   a. 50%
   b. 30%
   c. 0%
   d. 20%

10. An example of a pathological change in a patient which requires an increase in technique is:

    a. osteoporosis
    b. ascites
    c. pneumothorax
    d. emphysema

11. The pathology below that would require a decrease in technical factors is:

    a. congestive heart failure
    b. pneumonia
    c. edema
    d. osteomyelitis

12. A patient is being radiographed as a follow-up for a wrist fracture wearing a fiberglass cast to stabilize the fracture. To optimally expose the radiograph, the radiographer should:

    a. increase kVp 15% to ensure adequate penetration
    b. increase mAs to account for the cast's increased absorption of photons
    c. use the same PA wrist technique for a patient without a cast
    d. remove the cast to eliminate its superimposition over the anatomy; this also allows a typical PA wrist technique to be set

13. Which exam/anatomy below typically requires a decreased technique for optimal visualization of a foreign body?

    a. a barium-coated esophagus
    b. soft tissue neck
    c. lateral lumbar spine
    d. tibia to rule out osteopetrosis

14. The contrast media that would produce greater radiolucency of a structure when used during a radiographic exam would be:

    a. air
    b. water
    c. barium
    d. iodine

15. The most appropriate rule to apply for a corrective technique if a pelvis radiograph exhibits too low of density, no bony trabeculae are visible, and it is impossible to "see through" the part would be the:

    a. 30% rule for mAs
    b. 15% rule for kVp
    c. the 4 to 5 cm rule
    d. the 2 kVp rule

16. The advantages of an optimal kVp technique system include:

    1. Consistent contrast
    2. Adequate penetration of the part being imaged
    3. Radiographs of the highest contrast possible

    a. 1, 2
    b. 1, 3
    c. 2, 3
    d. 1, 2, 3

17. One of the advantages of a variable kVp-fixed mAs technique chart is:

    a. lower patient doses due to lower mAs used
    b. adequate penetration of the part is ensured
    c. the elimination of caliper use to measure patient thickness
    d. that once it is developed, the same chart can be used for all the x-ray units in a department

18. Based on comparative anatomy principles, identify the anatomical structure below that would probably employ a technique similar to an AP lumbar spine.

    a. AP knee
    b. PA hand
    c. AP abdomen
    d. PA chest

19. According to optimum kVp principles, which technique below would be the best starting point for an AP knee?

    a. 120 kVp at 3.2 mAs
    b. 70 kVp at 7.5 mAs
    c. 55 kVp at 1.2 mAs
    d. 80 kVp at 80 mAs

20. To develop a fixed kVp-variable mAs technique chart, the most appropriate rule to apply is the:

    a. 30% rule for mAs
    b. 15% rule for kVp
    c. the 4 to 5 cm rule
    d. the 2 kVp rule

21. The advantages of developing and using technique charts are:

    1. More consistent image quality
    2. Fewer repeat exposures
    3. Increased patient satisfaction

    a. 1, 2
    b. 1, 3
    c. 2, 3
    d. 1, 2, 3

22. Which of the following is NOT a step in technique chart development?

    a. have the radiologist(s) select the most optimal image(s)
    b. expose phantom images
    c. apply the 30% rule for patient thickness changes
    d. perform clinical trials on patients

23. Using variable kVp principles, if the original technique for an AP elbow exam is 65 kVp at 6 mAs and the patient measures 6 cm, what technique should be listed for a 10-cm AP elbow?

    a. 65 kVp at 12 mAs
    b. 65 kVp at 9 mAs
    c. 73 kVp at 6 mAs
    d. 73 kVp at 12 mAs

24. What new technique should be set to improve an AP hip radiograph that exhibits inadequate density and is inadequately penetrated if the original technique was 68 kVp at 20 mAs?

    a. 78 kVp at 20 mAs
    b. 78 kVp at 10 mAs
    c. 68 kVp at 40 mAs
    d. 68 kVp at 10 mAs

25. Generally, in order to maintain density and the exposure to the IR, as patient thickness increases:

    a. mAs should decrease
    b. mAs should increase
    c. kVp should increase
    d. kVp should decrease

26. Which exam below would be more likely to have a technique setting of 100 kVp?

    a. any iodine-based contrast media exam
    b. lateral vertebral column
    c. large extremities
    d. double-contrast barium enema

27. Using fixed kVp principles, if the original technique for an AP shoulder exam is 72 kVp at 12.5 mAs and the patient measures 16 cm, what technique should be listed for a 12-cm AP shoulder?

    a. 64 kVp at 12.5 mAs
    b. 64 kVp at 25 mAs
    c. 72 kVp at 25 mAs
    d. 72 kVp at 6 mAs

28. To correctly measure a patient, the caliper should be placed:

    a. to match the OID level
    b. at the fulcrum level
    c. level with the central ray entrance point
    d. to measure the thinnest and thickest portion of the anatomy

29. What technique system is being used if a technologist measures the proximal forearm, doubles it, and adds this value to a baseline value of 30 for the kVp setting?

    a. variable kVp-fixed mAs
    b. flexible mAs-flexible kVp
    c. comparative anatomy
    d. fixed kVp-variable mAs

30. What imaging situation below will reduce the number of photons reaching the image receptor, requiring a change in technique?

    a. the use of a negative contrast medium
    b. a hypersthenic patient
    c. the presence of an osteolytic lesion
    d. performing a chest exam on a 3-year-old patient

Labeling

1. Evaluate the patients shown. Identify each body habitus type. Below each type, describe the general build of this body habitus type and its approximate percentage of occurrence in the patient population.

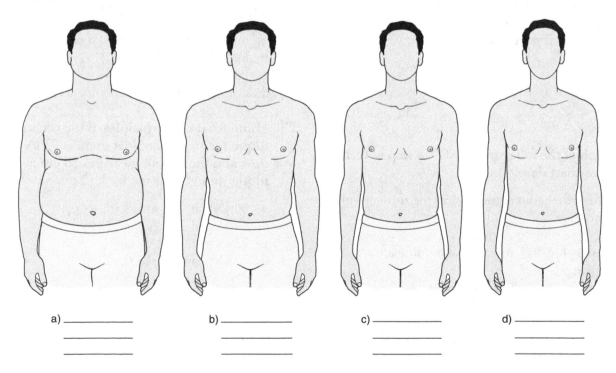

a) _____
   _____
   _____

b) _____
   _____
   _____

c) _____
   _____
   _____

d) _____
   _____
   _____

2. Complete the table indicating the optimal kVp for the anatomical region listed.

Region	Optimal kVp Range
Small extremities (hand, foot, etc.)	_____
Iodine-based contrast media exams	_____
Large extremities (shoulder, knee, etc.)	_____
Skull	_____
Abdomen and ribs	_____
AP vertebral column	_____
Lateral vertebral column	_____
Barium exams (double contrast)	_____
Chest	_____
Barium exams (single contrast)	_____

3. Complete the table providing the missing technical factors for a 19-cm and 23-cm pelvis using variable kVp and fixed mAs principles.

VARIABLE kVp-FIXED mAs PELVIS

Part Thickness	Optimal kVp	mAs
15 cm	80	20
19 cm	—	—
23 cm	—	—

4. Complete the table providing the missing technical factors for a 19-cm and 23-cm pelvis using fixed kVp and variable mAs principles.

FIXED kVp-VARIABLE mAs PELVIS

Part Thickness	Optimal kVp	mAs
15 cm	80	20
19 cm	—	—
23 cm	—	—

Crossword Puzzle

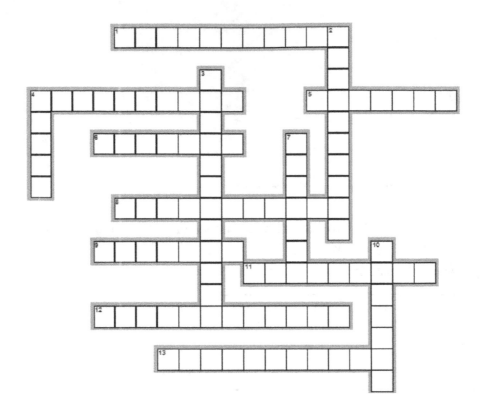

Across

1. A patient who is tall and slender would be classified as this type of body habitus
4. Type of cast material that requires no technique factor change
5. 70 kVp is the _____ kVp setting for large extremities; ensures adequate penetration for the part being imaged
6. Device to measure patient thickness
8. Term used to describe tissue that allows x-ray photons to travel through tissue with less attenuation
9. Type of test image prior to clinical trials to check for technique accuracy
11. Direction of technique change if soft tissue exam is performed
12. Body habitus type where patient thickness is greater than normal
13. _____ Anatomy: Technique principle that states that similar techniques may be used on different body parts if they have similar thicknesses and their tissue composition is similar

Down

2. Principle of technique that states, "No amount of mAs can ever _____ for kVp that is too low."
3. Subtractive disease process causing bone loss
4. Type of technique chart where kVp does not change and mAs is varied; ____ kVp
7. Average body habitus type
10. Additive disease process due to accumulation of fluid in the abdomen

Automatic Exposure Control

18

1. All of the following are primary advantages of automatic control systems EXCEPT:

   a. less uniform results
   b. less affected by line fluctuation
   c. less patient dose
   d. less repeat radiographs

2. The most critical factor in obtaining diagnostic quality images using an AEC circuit is the use of accurate:

   a. positioning/centering
   b. focal spot size
   c. side markers
   d. backup time

3. In the traditional phototiming automatic exposure control systems:

   a. there is only one large detector
   b. photomultiplier tubes or photodiodes are used
   c. the detectors are placed between the patient and the IR
   d. remnant x-rays are converted to a laser raster pattern

4. When AEC systems are used, the technical factor no longer set or controlled by the technologist is:

   a. kVp
   b. mA
   c. time
   d. SID

5. When utilizing the AEC, changing the mA from 100 to 300 will result in:

   a. more density
   b. less contrast
   c. a shorter exposure time
   d. less distortion

6. In most modern AEC systems, the detectors are composed of:

   a. photodiodes
   b. a gaseous substance
   c. silicon or selenium
   d. tungsten

7. When would it be appropriate for a technologist to note the mAs readout when an exposure is made using an automatic exposure control device?

   a. during technical factor selection
   b. during the prep phase of the exposure
   c. immediately after the exposure is made
   d. prior to releasing the patient

8. The purpose of the backup timer in an automatic exposure control system is to:

   a. increase the exposure time
   b. allow the ion chambers enough time to respond to the remnant radiation
   c. provide the technologist with a mechanism to verify the actual mAs of the exposure
   d. prevent excessive exposure by terminating the exposure in case of technologist error

9. **If the minimum response time of an AEC unit is longer than the exposure time needed for a diagnostic quality radiograph, which of the following will best describe the final radiograph?**

   a. density will be too high due to the longer exposure time
   b. no density will be present on the film because the unit is not able to engage to even start the exposure time needed
   c. density will be too low, because the unit will shut off too soon
   d. the unit will automatically shut off at 1.5 times the necessary exposure once the backup time is reached

10. **A radiograph exposed using AEC comes out 50% denser than it should be. For the repeat, set the density knob to:**

    a. N
    b. −1
    c. −2
    d. +1

11. **The expected exposure for an AP knee is 75 kVp at 10 mAs (100 mA and 0.1 s). To ensure adequate exposure during an AEC exposure, the technologist should set:**

    a. the backup technique at 20 mAs (100 mA and 0.2 s)
    b. the density (intensity) control at −2
    c. the backup timer at 5000 ms
    d. the minimum response time to 1 ms

12. **A manual technique rather than an AEC exposure would be required for which of the radiographic exams below?**

    a. a PA and lateral chest x-ray on a patient with a cough
    b. a standing knee on a patient for a postsurgical knee replacement
    c. a KUB and upright abdomen on a 14-year-old male patient with a 22 cm abdominal thickness
    d. an AP pelvis on a 57-year-old slender female patient with a shoulder replacement

13. **While performing an abdomen examination in the erect position using an automatic exposure control unit, you use 72″ rather than 40″ SID (assume a nonfocused grid). The radiograph will be:**

    a. underexposed
    b. overexposed
    c. acceptable
    d. mottled

14. **After performing two erect views of a shoulder using an automatic exposure control, you place the image receptor on the tabletop for the axillary view with no other changes to the control panel. After positioning the patient for the axillary, what is likely to occur?**

    a. no exposure to the image receptor and the backup timer alarm will go off
    b. overexposure to the image receptor and the backup timer alarm will go off
    c. the exposure will be acceptable because the AEC detectors will automatically adjust the time needed
    d. overexposure because the image receptor is on the tabletop and the AEC detector is only used for exposures using the bucky

15.

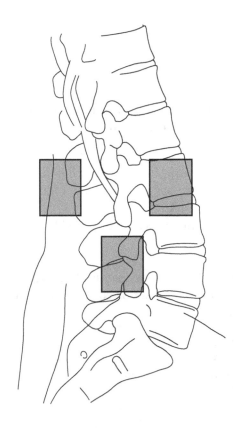

Evaluate the illustration and determine the quality of the resulting radiograph:

    a. the radiograph will be underexposed
    b. the radiograph will be overexposed
    c. the radiograph will be acceptable
    d. not enough information to tell

16. Which portion of the x-ray circuit are the automatic exposure control ion chambers connected to?

    a. secondary; step-up transformer
    b. filament; rheostat
    c. secondary; anode
    d. primary; timer

17. To obtain the appropriate amount of exposure during an AEC exposure:

    a. the thickest portion of the anatomy should be centered over the chamber(s)
    b. the backup timer should be set to 5000 ms
    c. the center ion chamber should be selected for every exposure
    d. the kVp needs to be at least 60 kVp or higher

18. An image taken using the AEC indicates underexposure and inadequate penetration. To correct this error for the repeat exposure, the technologists should:

    a. select a longer backup timer so that the AEC does not terminate the exposure prematurely
    b. select a lower ma so that the time is longer
    c. select a higher kVp setting using the 15% rule
    d. check to make sure the minimum response time is functioning before the next exposure

19. When using the AEC in conjunction with a digital imaging system, how would the radiographic image be affected if a 14 × 17″ field size is used on an AP cervical spine?

    a. the radiograph will be overexposed due to excessive fog
    b. the radiograph will be underexposed and quantum mottle may be present
    c. the radiograph will be acceptable
    d. no exposure will occur because the minimum response time will be too short

20. The most appropriate ion chamber selection for AP bilateral standing knees would be:

    a. the center cell only
    b. the two side cells
    c. one side cell and one center cell
    d. all three cells

21. Which of the exams below would be likely to use all three ion chambers during an AEC exposure?

    a. PA chest
    b. oblique lumbar spine
    c. AP abdomen
    d. PA wrist

22. Which of the following items would be found on an automatic exposure control technique chart?

    1. Backup time
    2. Ion chamber selection
    3. mAs readout

    a. 1, 2
    b. 1, 3
    c. 2, 3
    d. 1, 2, 3

23. All of the following are advantages of Anatomically Programmed Radiography (APR) EXCEPT:

    a. the radiographer can quickly set the exposure factors for a procedure
    b. eliminates the need for manual technique corrections
    c. it has streamlined the operator's control panel
    d. the correct AEC ion chambers are automatically selected

24. In the list below, identify the item that is not associated with technique factor selection:

    a. fixed kVp, variable mAs
    b. automatic exposure control
    c. anatomically controlled radiography
    d. all of these are technique selection systems

25. The set of circumstances below where AEC and digital imaging systems can be used to advantage are:

    a. selecting the center cell for a PA chest, allowing automatic rescaling to correct the exposure appearance
    b. AP portable chests, using double the time to ensure adequate exposure
    c. ensuring that the intensity controls are activated for each exposure
    d. the ability to use the identical cell selection for an AP hip and the frogleg lateral hip

For Questions 26 to 30, evaluate the automatic exposure control circumstances to determine if the radiograph will be/have:

    a. overexposed
    b. underexposed
    c. acceptable exposure

26. _____ Density control of −2 not changed from prior patient

27. _____ Table bucky selected instead of chest bucky for an AP shoulder

28. _____ Backup timer not set to match a large body habitus

29. _____ Center cell selected for an AP lumbar spine

30. _____ Gonad shield placed over the anatomy and the detector

Labeling

1. Complete the table indicating the correct detector selection for each procedure/projection.

Procedure	Projection	kVp	mA	Detector(s)	Density Control	SID and Notes
Chest	PA/AP	110–125	200		N	72″
	Lateral	110–125	200		N	72″
Ribs above diaphragm	AP/Obl	70	300		N	40″
Ribs below diaphragm	AP	70–80	400		N	40″
KUB	AP	80	400		N	40″
Pelvis	AP	80–85	400		N	40″
Hip	AP/Lat	80–85	400		+2	40″ *Medial and/or center
Lumbar spine	AP/Obl	75–85	400		N	40″
	Lat	80–90	400		N	40″
	L1/S1	85–95	400		N	40″
Thoracic spine	AP	75–85	300		N	40″
	Lat	80–90	400		N	40″ Breathing
Swimmers C/T	Lat	80–95	400		N	40″
Cervical spine	AP/odontoid	75–85	150		N	40″
	Obl/Lat	75–85	150		N	72″
Skull (sinus) (facial bones)	PA/Caldwell	70–80	150		N	40″
	Waters	70–80	150		N	40″
	Townes	70–80	150		N	40″
	Lateral	70–80	150		N	40″
Shoulder	AP	70–85	200		N	40″
Knee	AP/Obl/Lat	70–85	200		N	40″

Crossword Puzzle

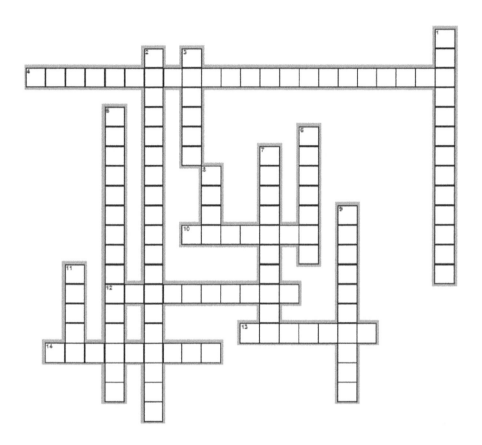

Across

4. _____ radiography; technique selection system that allows the technologist to economically select exposure factors by choosing the appropriate body part and view on the control panel
10. This is displayed immediately after an AEC exposure is taken and allows the technologist to know the actual exposure factors used: mAs _____
12. Most AEC systems have a configuration of three of these; _____ chamber
13. The location of the ion chambers in most AEC devices; _____ the patient and the image receptor
14. AEC devices are not recommended for use with this class of patients because they may be too small to fully cover at least one ionization chamber

Down

1. This occurs when the AEC device shuts off too soon, such as when the thickest part is not centered over an ion chamber
2. Time needed for an AEC unit to complete an exposure; as short as 1 ms (three words)
3. _____ time; this should usually be set so that it is two times longer than the expected needed exposure
5. _____ tube; AEC device that converts light to electricity
6. This AEC control allows a technologist to increase or decrease the preset exposure, usually in 25% increments
7. Solid state version of a PM tube
8. Technique factor controlled by the AEC during an exposure
9. Surgically implanted metal artifact commonly found in the hip or knee; typically not imaged well using AEC devices
11. Typical number of ion chambers in an AEC system

PART IV

Digital Imaging and Processing

19

Basic Principles of Digital Imaging

1. Some advantages of digital imaging over conventional screen/film radiography include:

   1. Immediate visualization of the image
   2. Ability to adjust the image postexposure
   3. Highest spatial resolution possible

   a. 1, 2
   b. 1, 3
   c. 2, 3
   d. 1, 2, 3

2. The H & D curve for digital imaging is linear rather than S shaped because:

   a. more line pairs per millimeter can be imaged
   b. larger field of views (FOV) are possible
   c. radiographic images are displayed in matrices, rather than analog
   d. of a wider dynamic range

3. A digital image is made up of:

   a. a pixel of matrices
   b. a matrix of pixels
   c. a vortex of pixels
   d. a matrix of vortices

4. Which matrix size has the smallest pixels?

   a. 128 × 128
   b. 256 × 256
   c. 512 × 512
   d. 1,024 × 1,024

5. What is the pixel size in millimeters of a 256 matrix with a 25-cm field of view?

   a. 0.1
   b. 1.0
   c. 10
   d. 100

6. What is the pixel size in millimeters of a 512 matrix with a 30-cm field of view?

   a. 0.06
   b. 0.6
   c. 6.0
   d. 60

7. What is the pixel size in millimeters of a 256 matrix with a 15-cm field of view?

   a. 0.06
   b. 0.6
   c. 6.0
   d. 60

8. **The field of view (FOV) best describes:**

    a. the number of pixels in a matrix
    b. the imaging plane that is best demonstrated
    c. how much of the patient is imaged in a matrix
    d. the use of multiformat cameras to display multiple images

9. **If the field of view remains unchanged and the matrix size increases, the spatial resolution will be:**

    a. improved
    b. degraded
    c. constant

10. **If the field of view increases and the matrix size is unchanged, pixel size will:**

    a. increase
    b. decrease
    c. remain unchanged also

11. **Which of the following will allow more line pairs/mm to be imaged?**

    a. using a smaller matrix
    b. increasing the number of pixels
    c. increasing the bit depth
    d. using a higher-frequency signal

12. **The number of shades of gray that can be demonstrated in a digital image is affected by:**

    a. matrix size
    b. bit depth
    c. field of view
    d. data compression

13. **Contrast resolution describes:**

    a. the maximum separation of two objects that can be distinguished as separate objects on the image
    b. the minimum density difference between two tissues that can distinguish separate tissues
    c. the maximum density difference between two tissues that can be distinguished as separate tissues
    d. the minimum separation of two objects that can be distinguished as separate objects on the image

14. **The amount of luminance of an image or light displayed by a monitor is termed:**

    a. brightness
    b. density
    c. contrast
    d. spatial frequency

15. **The anatomical structures that would cause the greatest degree of x-ray photon attenuation and image brightness would be those that are:**

    a. radiolucent
    b. radioactive
    c. radiopaque
    d. radiodense

16. **The window width control is used to alter image:**

    a. contrast
    b. brightness
    c. signal-to-noise ratio
    d. resolution

17. **The window level control is used to alter image:**

    a. contrast
    b. brightness
    c. resolution
    d. signal-to-noise ratio

18. **If the window width control is opened wider:**

    a. the image will appear denser
    b. overall brightness will increase
    c. the image's edges will appear sharper
    d. more gray shades will be available

19. **Spatial detail in a digital imaging system would be improved MOST by:**

    a. increasing the window width
    b. decreasing the window level
    c. increasing the number of pixels
    d. decreasing the flux gain of the photomultiplier tube

20. **If a pixel has a bit depth of 8, this means that the pixel:**

    a. is able to resolve 8 lp/mm
    b. can produce 256 shades of gray
    c. the pixel size is 0.8 mm
    d. contains 8 bytes of information

21. **If an anatomical structure is smaller than one pixel:**

    a. only two shades of gray are possible
    b. the structure will not be visualized
    c. postexposure image manipulation is not possible
    d. greater line pairs per millimeter measurements are obtained

22. **Calculate the spatial frequency of an imaging system if the pixel size is 0.15 mm:**

    a. 0.30 lp/mm
    b. 1.5 lp/mm
    c. 3.33 lp/mm
    d. 6.67 lp/mm

23. **If pixel density is increased, the image will have/display:**

    a. increased spatial resolution
    b. decreased spatial resolution
    c. increased contrast resolution
    d. decreased contrast resolution

24. **If pixel pitch is increased, the image will have/display:**

    a. increased spatial resolution
    b. decreased spatial resolution
    c. increased contrast resolution
    d. decreased contrast resolution

25. **Which of the following image quality changes is undesirable?**

    a. increased spatial resolution
    b. increased contrast resolution
    c. increased image noise
    d. increased image matrix size

26. **If a high degree of quantum mottle is noted on an image, the most appropriate solution to correct this exposure error would be to:**

    a. raise the window level higher
    b. choose a larger pixel size
    c. repeat the exposure using a higher mAs
    d. have the patient remove their jewelry for the next exposure

27. **In general, as image noise increases:**

    a. brightness increases
    b. contrast decreases
    c. sharpness increases
    d. gray scale decreases

28. **Any unwanted information on an image is the definition for:**

    a. artifacts
    b. penumbra
    c. image fog
    d. pixel loss

29. **Which of the following is a contributor to image noise?**

    1. Scatter radiation
    2. Plus densities
    3. Minus densities

    a. 1, 2
    b. 1, 3
    c. 2, 3
    d. 1, 2, 3

30. **The use of high-resolution monitors:**

    a. promotes the visibility of anatomical structures
    b. minimizes the appearance of quantum mottle
    c. permits the use of increased mAs values
    d. limits the postprocessing of a digital image

Labeling

1. Complete the remaining pixel address designations in the image matrix.

COLUMNS

	1	2	3	4	5
1	1-1	2-1	3-1	4-1	5-1
2	1-2				
3	1-3				
4	1-4				
5	1-5				

ROWS

2. Evaluate the three lighthouse images. Based on their appearance, place them in order of their matrix sizes, with "1" being the smallest matrix and "3" being the largest.

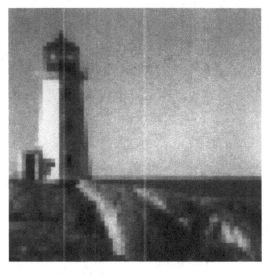

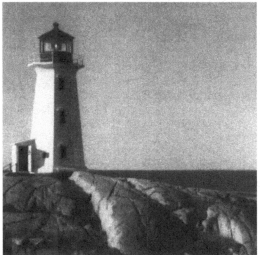

_____   _____

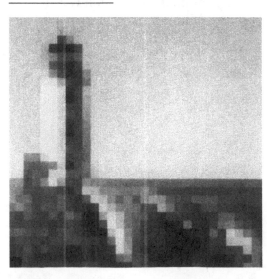

_____

3. Complete the table describing the relationships between field of view, matrix size, pixel size, and spatial resolution.

FOV	Matrix Size	Pixel Size	Spatial Resolution
Increases	_____	_____	_____
Decreases	_____	_____	_____
Remains constant	_____	_____	_____
Remains constant	_____	_____	_____

4. Evaluate the three lighthouse images. Based on their appearance, place them in order of their bit depth, with "1" being the lowest bit depth and "3" being the highest bit depth.

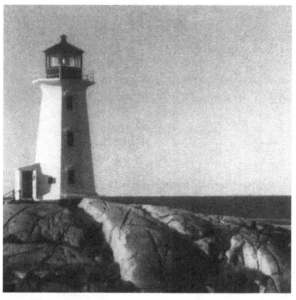

_____

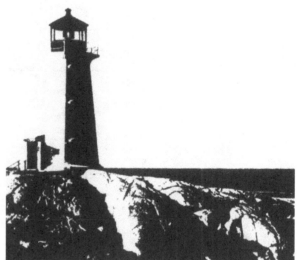

_____

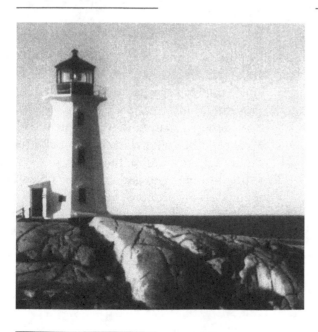

_____

Crossword Puzzle

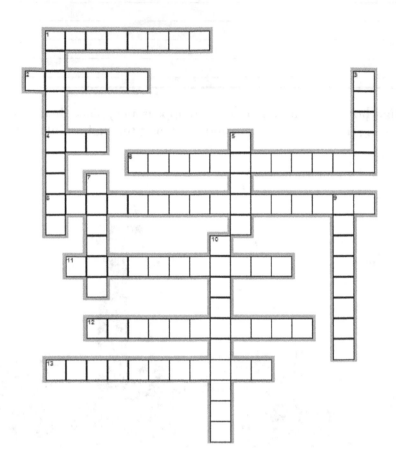

Across

1. Calculated using the formula, 2^n; reports the number of gray shades available (two words)
2. Language used by computers
4. The minimum number of pixels needed to image one line pair
6. The ability to detect and display a large range of radiographic densities: a wide _____ _____ (two words)
8. Formula to calculate this is 1/2 (PS); determines the number of line pairs that can be resolved if the pixel size is known (two words)
11. Postprocessing function that alters image contrast or gray scale (two words)
12. Postprocessing function that alters image brightness (two words)
13. Portion of the collimated field that contains the anatomy and displayed on the monitor (three words)

Down

1. Amount of luminance an image displays on a monitor
3. Image quality constituted of unwanted or useless background information
5. Each cell in a matrix; short for "picture element"
7. Array of cells arranged in columns and rows
9. _____ resolution; the ability of a system to distinguish between and/or display objects that attenuate x-ray photons differently
10. The distance or spacing from the middle of one pixel to the middle of an adjacent pixel (two words)

Capturing the Digital Image

20

1. One of the advantages of digital imaging is:

   a. several visual cues are present that indicate over- or underexposure of the image
   b. the image can be easily sent to remote locations
   c. the image is permanently fixed, preventing postexposure tampering
   d. it represents a continuous and analog range of signal

2. The active layer in the photostimulable phosphor of a CR imaging plate is typically made of:

   a. calcium tungstate
   b. rare earth materials
   c. amorphous selenium
   d. barium fluorohalide

3. Which of the following layers in a computed radiography cassette serves to ground the plate and reduce static electricity?

   a. radiolucent front
   b. lead foil back
   c. felt lining
   d. phosphor layer

4. The purpose of europium in the photostimulable phosphor is to:

   a. convert x-rays to light
   b. convert light to an electric signal
   c. trap metastable electrons
   d. return excited electrons to their ground state

5. If the phosphor layer in a CR system is considered turbid, this means that:

   a. it is arranged in columns and rows
   b. it has been painted on to a support such as glass
   c. it is a slower speed class, requiring higher technique factors
   d. it is randomly arranged across the support layer

6. The device that is needed to allow computer processing of an analog signal is a/an:

   a. ADC
   b. PSP
   c. AMA
   d. PACS

7. Data compression:

   a. results in faster image processing
   b. produces faster transmission times
   c. requires less storage space
   d. does all of the above

8. Direct radiography eliminates the need for the _____ because the image is captured by multiple sensors that create an image signal immediately.

   a. image receptor cassette
   b. monitor
   c. automatic brightness control (ABC)
   d. photomultiplier tube

9. In order to view a digital image that has been exposed on a phosphor plate cassette, what "processing" equipment is needed?

   a. an automatic processor
   b. a barcode-enabled RIS
   c. a radiographic film scanner
   d. a laser reader

10. The "latent image" in a CR imaging plate is stored by the:

    a. photomultiplier tube
    b. analog-to-digital converter (ADC)
    c. sensitivity speck
    d. trapped electrons in the phosphor

11. In direct radiography, remnant radiation is converted into an electric signal by:

    a. barium fluorohalide crystals
    b. an electron gun
    c. magnesium oxide
    d. amorphous selenium

12. The component of a direct flat panel detector that is responsible for absorbing electrons and generating the subsequent electrical charges to the image processor is the:

    a. photostimulable phosphor
    b. thin-film transistor
    c. light shield layer
    d. conductive layer

13. The device that converts the light emitted by an exposed PSP in a computed radiography (CR) reader to an electric signal is the:

    a. photodiode
    b. scanning laser
    c. thin-film transistor
    d. digital-to-analog converter

14. Before a computed radiography imaging plate can be reused, it must be:

    a. stored in a darkened room for 24 hours
    b. erased with high-intensity light
    c. scanned with an electron gun
    d. recharged

15. After exposure, the remaining steps for acquiring a computed radiography image, in order, are:

    a. stimulation, reading, and erasing
    b. charging, storing, and dumping
    c. scanning, quantization, and cleaning
    d. developing, fixing, and filing

16. The laser in a CR reader:

    a. releases a blue high-intensity light that is sent to an ADC
    b. scans the exposed phosphor in a raster pattern
    c. is used to power the barcode scanner of the workstation
    d. eliminates any residual fog or ghosting

17. The system responsible for opening the IP and transporting the exposed phosphor through the CR reader is the _____ system.

    a. transit
    b. computer drive
    c. mechanical
    d. gateline

18. In a direct radiography system, a charge-coupled device is used to:

    a. detect x-ray photons, converting them to a digital signal
    b. detect and convert light photons to a digital signal
    c. stimulate the exposed plate to emit bright white light
    d. ensure that the signal is not dumped prematurely

19. In indirect capture, the scintillation device is commonly composed of:

    a. cesium iodide
    b. amorphous selenium
    c. fiberoptic bundles
    d. fluorohalide

20. The functional unit of a direct radiography flat panel is a:

    a. pixel
    b. cell
    c. dexel
    d. CCD tile

21. **Flat-field correction is:**

    a. a postprocessing function to manipulate the image's appearance
    b. the systematic dumping of information line-by-line in a DR system
    c. a software interpolation that fills in information due to seams in the panel
    d. part of the annual maintenance for a painted a-Si glass panel

22. **The function of a thin-film transistor in an indirect DR system is to:**

    a. serve as a switch that allows a capacitor to collect charge during exposure
    b. convert the light from the scintillator to a digital signal
    c. continuously apply a negative charge to the DR panel
    d. prevent moisture from reaching the scintillating material

23. **All of the following statements are true regarding dexels EXCEPT:**

    a. they are composed of a photodetector phase and electronic components
    b. they require several CCDs to be tiled together in order to work
    c. they are only about 80% efficient
    d. the collection element is typically amorphous silicon

24. **The image receptor system that is typically constructed with amorphous selenium sandwiched between two charged electrodes best describes which imaging system?**

    a. computed radiography
    b. automatic exposure control
    c. direct capture
    d. indirect capture

25. **The latent image of a direct capture DR image is formed by:**

    a. amorphous selenium "holes"
    b. cesium iodide scintillation points
    c. electrons trapped in the conduction band
    d. ionized silver atoms collected by the sensitivity speck

26. **After the exposure, the active matrix array (AMA):**

    a. emits visible light in response to remnant radiation
    b. controls the gatelines to ensure that the data are provided in sequential order
    c. interpolates the data from the unexposed datalines
    d. neutralizes the charge in each dexel prior to sending it to the ADC

27. **The electrical device responsible for collecting charge in a circuit is the:**

    a. capacitor
    b. fiberoptic bundle
    c. photodiode
    d. rheostat

28. **The three steps taken to convert a conventional radiographic film to a digital image include all of the following EXCEPT:**

    a. sampling
    b. quantization
    c. scintillation
    d. scanning

29. **Banding artifacts can result when:**

    a. the PSP is inadequately erased after exposure
    b. the number of photons reaching the IR is inadequate
    c. the mechanical system of a CR reader is defective
    d. an inadequate number of pixels were sampled during scanning

30. **The process of assigning number values to each pixel in proportion to the energy received best describes:**

    a. sampling
    b. dumping
    c. ionization
    d. quantization

Labeling

1. Label each component in the digital imaging chain.

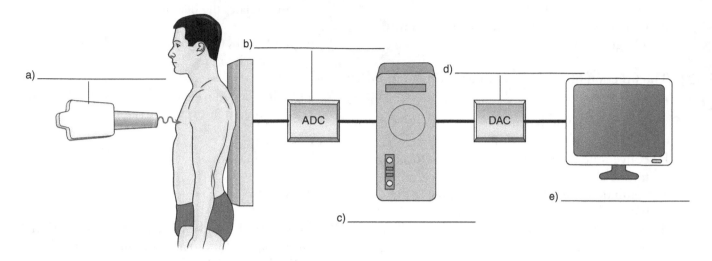

2. Identify the layers of the photostimulable phosphor.

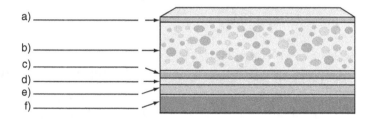

3. Label each charge-coupled device (CCD) component.

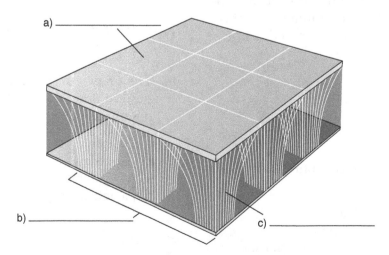

4. Fill-in-the blanks by identifying each component of a thin-film transistor (TFT) array.

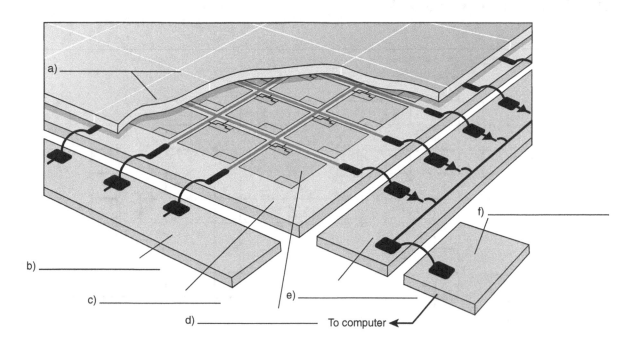

a) _____

b) _____

c) _____

d) _____ To computer

e) _____

f) _____

5. Identify each layer of a dexel in a direct capture flat panel detector.

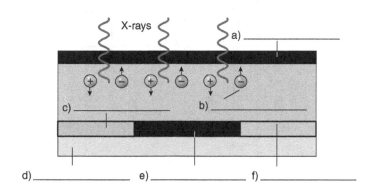

X-rays

a) _____

b) _____

c) _____

d) _____ e) _____ f) _____

Crossword Puzzle

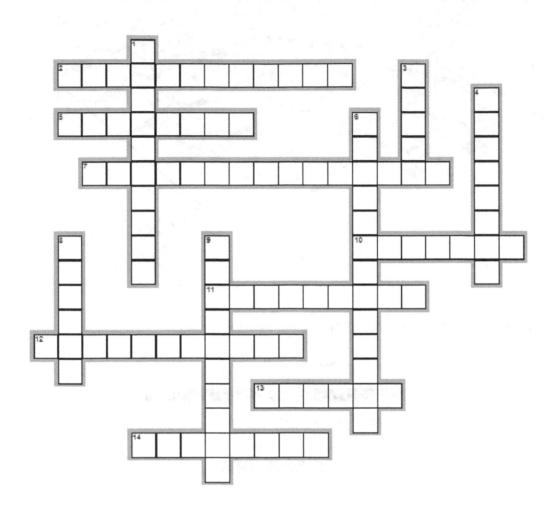

Across

2. The scintillation crystal commonly used in indirect capture DR (two words)
5. The photoconductor used in direct radiography systems
7. _____ phosphor; describes its ability to be excited by light
10. Step that clears an exposed IP for reuse using a bright white light
11. Denotes that crystals in the phosphor are randomly distributed
12. Collapses data into smaller files to promote faster transmission times
13. Pattern of lines formed by the laser in a CR reader
14. Barium fluorohalide is doped with this element

Down

1. A bundle of solid, light-conducting material (two words)
3. Term for "detector element"
4. During digitization, the process of detecting and measuring the exposure received by the detector
6. _____ device; converts light to an electrical signal when a DR system is used (two words)
8. Term that describes a continuously varying quantity or signal
9. Thin-film _____; switch that allows charge to be collected during a DR exposure

21

Digital Imaging Exposure Techniques

1. When developing exposure factors for a digital imaging system, which of the following factors no longer needs to be considered?

   a. body habitus of the patient
   b. ALARA
   c. optimal kVp settings
   d. all of these must still be considered

2. If a technologist fails to properly center over the appropriate automatic exposure control (AEC) cell, what undesirable results are likely to occur?

   a. underexposure and mottle
   b. overexposure and saturation
   c. underpenetration and histogram errors
   d. scatter fog and increased exposure index values

3. If a technologist fails to properly align the exposure field with a digital image receptor, what undesirable results are likely to occur?

   a. underexposure and mottle
   b. overexposure and saturation
   c. histogram errors and suboptimal EI values
   d. scatter fog and "ghosting"

4. The software function responsible for evaluating the collimated borders of an exposed imaging plate is called:

   a. algorithmic application
   b. exposure field recognition
   c. image equalization
   d. postprocessing

5. One of the problems identified with the technologist interface with digital imaging systems and technique selection is that:

   a. visual cues indicating over- or underexposure are no longer present on the image
   b. the image can be easily sent to remote locations
   c. kVp manipulation is severely limited compared to film/screen systems
   d. automatic exposure control systems cannot be used in tandem with digital systems

True/False: For Questions 6 to 10, determine if each statement is true or false with regard to digital imaging systems and optimal exposure factor selection. Answer A for true and B for false.

6. _____ The 15% rule can be used to adjust technique for changed patient thickness.

7. _____ Digital imaging systems are inherently mAs driven.

8. _____ The field size must be large enough so that at least 30% of the image receptor is exposed.

9. _____ It is recommended that all exposures be made using a minimum of 70 kVp.

10. _____ To avoid image mottle, expose all digital images without a grid whenever possible.

11. The practice of using higher exposure factors than needed to obtain a diagnostic radiograph is commonly referred to as:

    a. ALARA
    b. rounding up
    c. dose creep
    d. saturation

12. According to comparative anatomy principles, if a technologist has developed an acceptable technique for an AP L-spine, the technique for an AP pelvis would be:

    a. the same
    b. half the mAs
    c. 15% more kVp
    d. unrelated; it would actually be closer to an AP shoulder

13. Which of the following statements is true regarding kVp's role when using digital imaging systems?

    a. decreasing kVp significantly increases image contrast
    b. kVp ensures adequate penetration of the anatomy
    c. decreasing kVp decreases image brightness
    d. 80 kVp is now the recommended setting for virtually all exams

14. The quality that best describes digital imaging's ability to display a diagnostic radiograph even if the technical factors used are 400% greater than actually needed is exposure:

    a. latitude
    b. creep
    c. stabilization
    d. compensation

15. When an image is said to be "saturated," this means that:

    a. it has had inadequate time to dry
    b. image noise has exceeded an optimal level
    c. excessive overexposure has occurred
    d. the backup timer engaged during an AEC exposure

16. The factors responsible for the phenomena of dose creep when digital imaging systems are used include:

    1. Fear of mottle on the image
    2. No visible consequences for overexposure
    3. Speed class of CR/DR is 200 versus film/screen speed of 400

    a. 1, 2
    b. 1, 3
    c. 2, 3
    d. 1, 2, 3

17. When developing techniques for direct or computed radiography, the optimum kVp should generally be _____ compared to what is used in film/screen radiography.

    a. raised 10 kVp
    b. lowered 10 kVp
    c. raised 30 kVp
    d. lowered 30 kVp

18. If a department is converting from one imaging system to another, which of the following actions will need to be taken to ensure proper exposure levels are maintained?

    a. the grids must be removed or converted also
    b. the AEC will need to be recalibrated
    c. the SIDs will need to be rechecked
    d. the raster pattern will need to be doubled

19. A CR image appears "foggy," and the exposure indicator value indicates that a higher exposure than normal has reached the imaging plate. To prevent this from occurring on another image, the technologist should:

    a. note the EI value and use a correspondingly lower mAs on the next exposure
    b. check to make sure that she/he was centered over the appropriate AEC cells
    c. ensure that the anatomy and exposure field are aligned with the IR
    d. perform erasure of imaging plates on a daily or weekly basis

20. In order for multiple images to be performed on the same CR imaging plate, the anatomy must be centered and:

    a. separated with visible unexposed areas between each exposure
    b. imaged at right angles to each other
    c. with each projection imaged with a progressively lower technique to counteract the increased scatter production
    d. exposed using 15% less kVp since a grid will not be used

21. Exposure field recognition errors could occur in which circumstance outlined below?

    a. using more than 30 kVp than recommended for the part
    b. imaging anatomy diagonally on an imaging plate
    c. setting an inadequate backup time during AEC use
    d. activating all three cells during an AEC exposure

22. Which of the following is considered best practice with regard to setting techniques and/or evaluating images when digital imaging systems are used?

    a. increase mAs by two times for the next exposure if the image appears too bright on the monitor
    b. to avoid a repeat exposure due to image mottle, always increase mAs
    c. do not repeat an overexposed image if postprocessing can be used
    d. avoid collimating to ensure that all parts of the IR or detector array receive remnant radiation

23. If a grid is used in conjunction with a digital imaging system:

    a. a nongrid technique can be used
    b. technique can be unchanged from the department's previous film/screen techniques
    c. the same grid factor conversion formulas can be used as those used in film/screen
    d. it must be used for all exposures, including small extremities

24. When using a digital imaging system, the generally accepted range of kVps for pediatric patients is:

    a. 40 to 80
    b. 50 to 90
    c. 60 to 120
    d. 70 to 80

25. In general, regardless of the image receptor system used, _____ mAs can compensate for inadequate kVp.

    a. 100 times the
    b. 8 to 10 times the
    c. no amount of
    d. a low

Labeling

1. Evaluate the two H & D curves demonstrated in this illustration. Identify which curve represents film/screen and which curve represents a digital imaging system by filling in the blanks.

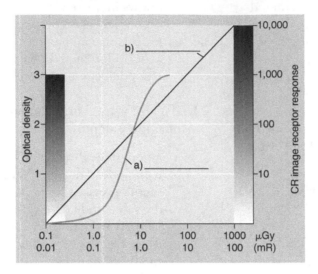

2. Fill-in-the blanks by identifying the image problem or potential problem demonstrated in each radiograph or diagram (on this and the next page) from the following choices: quantum mottle, histogram errors, image fog, and saturation.
   In the second blank line under each radiograph or illustration, state the primary cause of the problem identified.

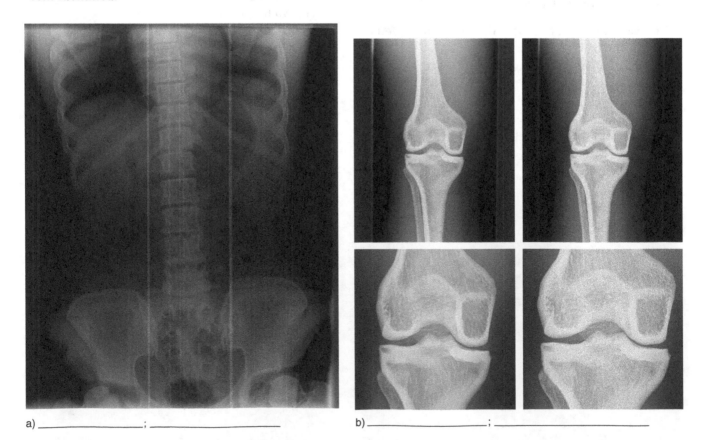

a) _____ ; _____   b) _____ ; _____

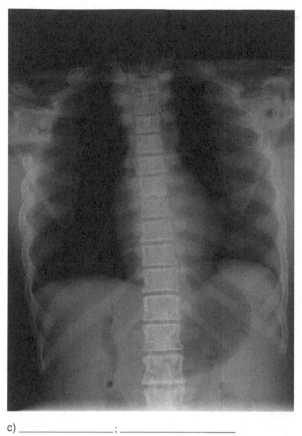

c) _____ ; _____

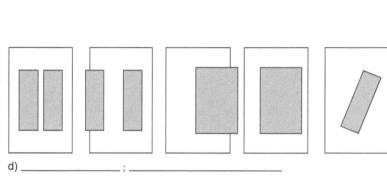

d) _____ ; _____

Crossword Puzzle

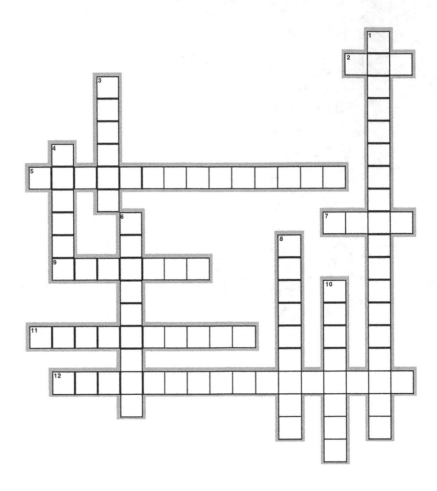

Across

2. The type of image noise that results if a CR imaging plate is left in an exam room while exposures are made
5. Windowing is an example of this function that allows manipulation of an image's brightness or contrast after exposure (two words or hyphenated)
7. Device that should be used in conjunction with an IR if the part thickness is more than 10 cm
9. Performing this action will prevent the appearance of fog on a CR image
11. Occurs when there is severe overexposure to the image receptor
12. This describes the appearance of the anatomy when kVp is too low and remnant radiation is unable to get through the part

Down

1. A method of technique factor selection that allows the technologist to use the same technique on different procedures due to their similar thicknesses and tissue composition (two words)
3. The minimum percentage of the IR that must be exposed to ensure adequate exposure and an acceptable EI value
4. A form of image noise that occurs when there is an inadequate number of photons exposing the IR; "quantum _____"
6. The undesirable practice of using more technique than is necessary to expose a radiograph (two words)
8. The graph generated by the computer that represents the range of pixel intensities in an image
10. The quality of CR/DR systems that allows visualization of anatomy even if the technique factor settings are more than 100% too high: "Exposure _____"

22

Digital Image Processing Operations

1. Which of the following is NOT a component of preprocessing?

   a. segmentation
   b. exposure field recognition
   c. low-pass filtering
   d. normalization

2. If a technologist fails to collimate during a digital imaging exposure, what undesirable image result could occur?

   a. quantum mottle
   b. exposure field recognition errors and altered exposure index values
   c. spatial distortion and a blurred image
   d. loss of the tail in the histogram and image inversion

3. A graph representing all of the image brightness values in an image is called a/an:

   a. mask
   b. spike
   c. algorithmic slope
   d. histogram

4. The software function responsible for evaluating the collimated borders of an exposed imaging plate is called:

   a. algorithmic application
   b. exposure field recognition
   c. image equalization
   d. postprocessing

5. Which of the following items best describes the spike or tail that is commonly present in an exposure histogram?

   a. density(ies) on the image that fall outside the actual anatomy
   b. it is used by the LUT to correct overexposure
   c. it defines the parameters of the expected exposure
   d. it dictates the final shape of the image histogram

6. The step in preprocessing that scans the imaging plate for the number and orientation of views is called:

   a. rescaling
   b. normalization
   c. segmentation
   d. annotation

7. **Which of the following could serve to skew histogram formation or analysis?**

   1. Prostheses
   2. Gonadal shielding
   3. Eliminating the graph's tail

   a. 1, 2
   b. 1, 3
   c. 2, 3
   d. 1, 2, 3

8. **A look-up table (LUT) would be used during which phase of image acquisition?**

   a. technique factor selection
   b. the partitioned pattern recognition phase
   c. image inversion
   d. histogram analysis

9. **The rescaling function during digital image acquisition serves to:**

   a. change the orientation of the image
   b. adjust image brightness to appear at optimal levels
   c. repair segmentation errors in a proportional manner
   d. increase the number of gray values available

10. **What effect does dynamic-range compression (DRC) have on the appearance of a digital image?**

    a. increased spatial resolution
    b. decreased image noise
    c. increased contrast
    d. decreased magnification

11. **Normalization plays what role in image acquisition?**

    a. aligns raw image data so that it resembles a conventional radiograph
    b. ensures the image is displayed in the correct orientation
    c. presets the average exposure settings
    d. creates data to be displayed in the unexposed area of the imaging plate

12. **During image acquisition, the component most responsible for the default appearance of the image is a/an:**

    a. ROI
    b. DRC
    c. ADC
    d. LUT

13. **To overcome or minimize the effect of a prosthesis in the exposure field, which type of LUT would most likely be used?**

    a. type 3
    b. type A-B
    c. global type
    d. bony type

14. **Which exposure situation would be the most likely to produce a histogram without a tail or spike?**

    a. exposure setting of < 69 kVp
    b. an exposure field that is placed diagonally on the IP
    c. the IP is completely covered by the exposure field and anatomy
    d. scatter fog present beyond the collimated borders of the exposure field

15. **The majority of the exposure data are processed by the computer using:**

    a. algorithms
    b. masking
    c. photodiodes
    d. CD drives

16. **Which statement is true with regard to post-processing?**

    a. it allows the technologist to electronically reduce the exposed field
    b. the image can be manipulated after exposure to please any viewer
    c. it prevents scatter radiation from creating image noise
    d. it describes the first era of digital imaging as film use decreased

17. The domains that can be altered to manipulate a digital image's appearance after exposure include:

    1. Magnetic
    2. Spatial
    3. Frequency

    a. 1,2
    b. 1, 3
    c. 2, 3
    d. 1, 2, 3

18. High-pass filtering would most affect which image quality?

    a. magnification
    b. contrast or gray scale
    c. spatial resolution or detail
    d. image brightness

19. The type of algorithm that may be used in the postprocessing phase that suppresses the low spatial frequencies to enhance the image is (the):

    a. subtractive type
    b. Fourier transform
    c. gradation curve
    d. dynamic-range compression

20. Edge enhancement functions are used to:

    a. sharpen a blurred image in the spatial domain by adjusting image frequency
    b. subtract out a blurred mask from the original image
    c. increase the contrast between the exposed and unexposed portions of the imaging plate
    d. decrease both noise and brightness levels of individual pixels

For Questions 21 to 25, match the operator adjustment tools with their function or intended result.

21. _____ Image inversion
22. _____ Annotation
23. _____ Magnification
24. _____ Windowing
25. _____ Image rotation

    a. Visually enlarges structures on the monitor
    b. Re-orients image horizontally or vertically
    c. Alters image brightness or gray scale
    d. Allows letters or numbers to be added
    e. Reverses the whites and blacks in an image

26. If a different look-up table (LUT) or the volume of interest (VOI) is changed by the technologist:

    a. the number of pixels in the image will change
    b. a different tissue type would be accentuated
    c. exposure latitude will change also
    d. the average gray scale curve will become steeper

27. Which of the following preprocessing steps would be the most likely to increase the appearance of image contrast?

    a. low-pass filtering
    b. normalization
    c. using dynamic-range compression
    d. applying a type 3 LUT

28. Which of the following situations would change the position of the exposure histogram?

    a. using an AEC exposure device in conjunction with a DR panel
    b. cropping the images prior to interpretation
    c. using twice the mAs needed for the exposure
    d. placing only one projection or view in the center of the IP

29. What is the significance of S1 and S2 in image acquisition processing?

    a. these serve as noise identifiers in the raw data and will ultimately be deleted during processing
    b. S1 is used for normal sampling; S2 is used to sample twice as much data
    c. S2 is subtracted from S1 during the rescaling process
    d. S1 and S2 are two points that define the area of the histogram the computer will analyze

30. A Type 2 LUT would be the most helpful for:

    a. compensating for a gonadal shield imaged in the exposure field
    b. placing a tail on the right side of the histogram
    c. counteracting anatomy that fills the entire image receptor
    d. applying a mask to the image to sharpen it

Labeling

1. Evaluate the histogram shown and label the anatomy that would typically be demonstrated in each of the blanks using S1 and S2 as a reference.

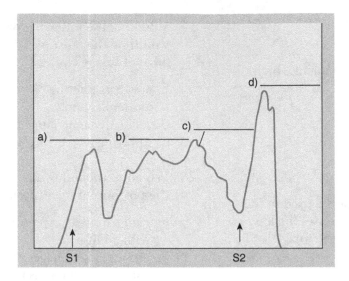

2. Fill-in-the blanks for each of the graphs identifying their spatial and frequency components.

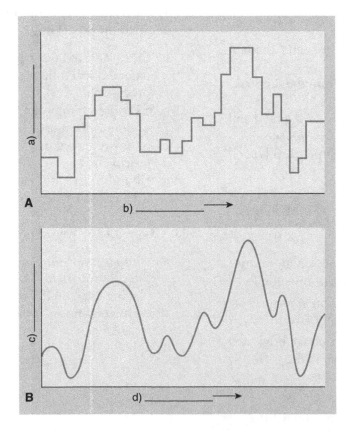

Crossword Puzzle

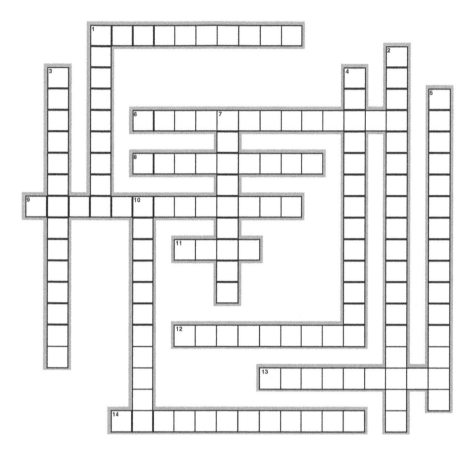

Across

1. Postprocessing step that allows the technologist to add letters or numbers to the image after exposure
6. Preprocessing step when the IR is scanned for collimation borders; _____ _____ recognition (two words)
8. A graph of the full range of the pixel brightness values in an image
9. Also called gradation; process that takes the raw data of an image and makes it appear as a conventional radiograph
11. The "spike" or portion of the histogram that represents the densities outside the anatomy
12. The process of adjusting the image to appear with normal brightness in the event of an under- or overexposure
13. Postprocessing step that reverses an image's appearance so that black appears white and vice versa: Image _____
14. Step in preprocessing when the imaging plate is scanned for the number and orientation of views

Down

1. A mathematical formula used to process image data
2. An adjustment to the brightness or contrast of an image by altering the exposure histogram to conform to the ideal reference histogram (two words)
3. All of the manipulation and adjustments to the digital image after corrections in the image acquisition stage
4. Also called image acquisition processing; takes place in the computer and corrects any flawed data
5. High-pass filtering; process that sharpens a blurred image by adjusting the frequency components (two words)
7. Low-pass filtering reduces both noise and brightness in an image
10. LUT; the reference histogram stored in the computer for each anatomical part and view (hyphen, two words)

23

Digital Exposure Indicators

1. Detective quantum efficiency (DQE) is used:

   a. to calculate the median average value of a central pixel
   b. to measure a phosphor's ability to convert x-ray energy to an output signal
   c. to determine an image's exposure index (EI) value after exposure
   d. as a measure of image receptor dose when DR detectors are used

2. Which of the following phosphors has the highest detective quantum efficiency?

   a. amorphous selenium
   b. silver bromide
   c. cesium iodide
   d. barium fluorobromide

3. In general, if an image receptor system has a high DQE:

   a. higher kVps should be used
   b. image noise will be increased
   c. more mAs should be used
   d. lower technical factors are required

4. The formula, SNR^2 output/SNR^2 input is used to:

   a. determine the exposure index value for CR IPs
   b. calculate the amount of shift needed between the exposure histogram and the LUT
   c. eliminate the electronic noise in the raw data
   d. calculate a system's detective quantum efficiency latitude

5. A device that would be found on a direct exposure system as an exposure indicator is a:

   a. photodiode
   b. DAP meter
   c. DQE calculator
   d. ADC EI writer

6. Which of the following would result in increased patient doses overall?

   a. using larger field sizes
   b. setting higher kVp techniques
   c. using longer SIDs
   d. reducing mAs values

7. In digital imaging systems, a numerical value is displayed with every image called an exposure indicator. This value is representative of the:

   1. Dose to the patient
   2. Dose to the IR
   3. Technique factors used

   a. 1, 2
   b. 1, 3
   c. 2, 3
   d. 1, 2, 3

8. Which of the following best describes the process used to derive most exposure index values?

   a. it is simply the dose (in mR) to the image receptor being reported
   b. the highest and lowest values in the exposure histogram are subtracted from each other and the difference is reported as the EI
   c. the degree of shift required to obtain the median pixel value of the exposure histogram to the LUT histogram is calculated
   d. by using the formula, $kVp \times ma \times time \times the_{log} 0.3$

9. The look-up table (LUT) is used during which phase of image acquisition?

   a. technique factor selection
   b. histogram analysis
   c. image inversion
   d. detector calibration

10. If the exposure index value exactly matches the manufacturer's quoted value, this means that:

   a. exposure factors and conditions were optimal
   b. the maximum acceptable dose to the IR was reached
   c. there was a 200 mm shift between the exposure histogram and the LUT
   d. there is likely to be quantum mottle present in the image

11. With regard to technique selection in digital imaging, which combination of factors below is recommended to properly expose a detector or IP and spare patient dose as much as possible?

   a. the lowest mAs setting available and 100+ kVp
   b. a high mAs with no more than 70 kVp
   c. a mAs setting of 20 with any kVp ranging from 40 to 80
   d. increased kVp and decreased mAs with no mottle present

12. In digital imaging, quantum mottle is due to:

   a. inadequate exposure to the IR
   b. overexposure to the patient
   c. excessive kVp settings and backscatter
   d. the phosphor make-up of the IR

For Questions 13 to 20, evaluate each statement with regard to exposure indicators to determine if each statement is true or false. Answer A for true and B for false.

13. _____ The EI values used in all digital imaging systems are uniform.

14. _____ Both mAs and kVp are equally important in image creation and the EI.

15. _____ Technique corrections and mottle prevention should only be made by changing mAs.

16. _____ If the image appears to diagnostic on the monitor, the EI value will be within range, also.

17. _____ Focal spot size, grids, and SID/OID remain as important exposure factors in digital imaging.

18. _____ If an exposure scale is inversely proportional, a low EI indicates that the exposure was too low, also.

19. _____ mAs no longer plays a role in the appearance of the image or histogram.

20. _____ The 15% rule for kVp can be applied as many as two times without altering contrast when digital imaging systems are used.

21. The manufacturers that use a proportional exposure index scale are:

   a. Fuji and Konica
   b. Agfa and Carestream
   c. GE and Siemens
   d. Philips and IEC

22. In a logarithmic exposure index scale, a change of 0.3 is equivalent to:

   a. a doubling of the exposure
   b. a 30% change in mAs
   c. a factor of 3 change in exposure
   d. a negligible change in exposure

23. When using Carestream equipment, the recorded exposure index is 2,020. Based on these data, the technologist should:

    a. repeat the image due to saturation
    b. lower the technique to one-half of the mAs and repeat the exposure
    c. increase the kVp 15% and repeat the exposure
    d. send the image to the radiologist for interpretation

24. An image exposed using Konica CR imaging plates has an S number of 400, and there is quantum mottle apparent throughout the anatomy. To correct these errors, select the best action below:

    a. window and level the image so that brightness and contrast appear optimal
    b. repeat the exposure, doubling the technique using the 15% rule
    c. repeat the exposure, halving the original mAs
    d. select another ROI, then window to alter brightness and contrast

25. The desirable exposure indicator value for an Alara CR system is:

    a. 2.0
    b. 200
    c. 2,000
    d. 3,000

26. The manufacturer who uses an EI derived from the average of two values: one from an AEC exposure and one from a central quarter field is:

    a. GE
    b. Siemens
    c. Philips
    d. Fuji

27. Images obtained from a Fuji system have S numbers in the 125 to 150 range and appear to have adequate brightness and contrast. Based on this information, the technologist should:

    a. not repeat the exposures and send to the radiologist for interpretation
    b. repeat the exposures doubling the mAs
    c. repeat the exposures increasing the kVp by 15%
    d. repeat the exposures, but only use one-half of the original mAs

28. The group that has recommended that all manufacturers begin to use standardized exposure indicators in the United States is the:

    a. NCRP
    b. ALARA
    c. AAPM
    d. ARRT

29. The term proposed by the International Electrotechnical Commission (IEC) for use across all manufacturers as an exposure indicator is:

    a. sensitivity number
    b. DICOM value
    c. exposure quantum
    d. deviation index/indices

30. Using the new exposure indicator system proposed by the IEC, if the value in the DICOM header is +1, this means that the exposure to the IR:

    a. was slightly overexposed but probably does not need to be repeated
    b. exactly matched the expected exposure conditions
    c. was slightly underexposed, and only needs repeating if mottle is present
    d. was outside the allowable range of exposure

Labeling

1. Evaluate the diagrams shown and their respective field sizes. Based on the 3 mrad per gram dose as illustrated, place the total dose per gram at the end of each row in the space provided. Based on your calculations, select the field size that delivers more dose per area.

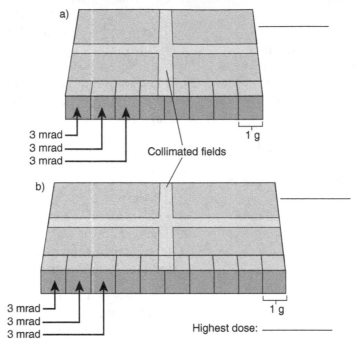

a) _____

3 mrad ——
3 mrad ——   Collimated fields
3 mrad ——

1 g

b) _____

3 mrad ——
3 mrad ——
3 mrad ——   Highest dose: _____

1 g

2. Complete the table by filling in the name of each manufacturer's exposure indicator, its symbol, and the type of EI scale it uses: proportional, logarithmic, or inversely proportional.

Manufacturer	Exposure Indicator	Symbol	Type of EI Scale
Agfa	_____	_____	_____
Alara CR	_____	_____	_____
Fuji	_____	_____	_____
General Electric	_____	_____	_____
CareStream	_____	_____	_____
Konica	_____	_____	_____
Philips	_____	_____	_____
Siemens	_____	_____	_____

Crossword Puzzle

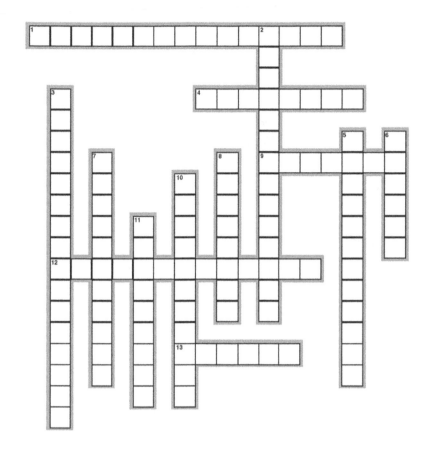

Across

1. Used as an indicator of exposure for direct radiography; calculated by multiplying the square of the field size times the dose (two words, hyphen)
4. The ability of an IR system to efficiently take a wide range of exposure values and convert them to an image: DQE _____
9. The relationship between two factors where one factor increases, but the other factor decreases
12. A value generated by the computer after comparing the exposure histogram with the reference histogram (two words)
13. Form of image noise that occurs when the exposure to the IR is insufficient

Down

2. The term recommended to be used by the IEC to represent more uniform exposure indicators such as −1, 0, +1 (two words)
3. The measure of a detector's or phosphor's ability to convert x-ray energy to an output signal (two words); _____ _____ Efficiency
5. The type of exposure indicator scale used where the technique used and the EI change at the same rate
6. The EI used by Agfa: Log _____
7. LUT; the reference histogram stored in the computer (two words, hyphen)
8. The DR phosphor with the highest DQE: amorphous _____
10. Type of exposure indicator scale that uses 0.3 to represent the doubling or halving of exposure
11. A graph representing all of the brightness values in an image

24

Digital Image Evaluation

1. Quantum mottle formation depends on:

   a. the K-shell absorption of the IR
   b. tube-bucky alignment
   c. the spatial resolution of the system
   d. the number of x-rays interacting with the IR

2. Which of the following items or criteria should be checked for on all digital images to ensure that the images are diagnostic in quality?

   1. Artifacts
   2. Pixel Brightness
   3. Exposure Index values

   a. 1, 2
   b. 1, 3
   c. 2, 3
   d. 1, 2, 3

3. Besides using an increased OID, the digital image can be made to appear magnified on a monitor. This can also cause the image to:

   a. lose spatial resolution and appear pixelated
   b. appear with higher contrast and reduced gray scale
   c. appear distorted and elongated
   d. be inadequately penetrated and mottled

4. Which of the following would result in increased signal-to-noise ratios and reduced patient doses overall?

   a. using larger field sizes
   b. setting higher kVp techniques
   c. Moiré effect
   d. setting higher mAs values

5. Any unwanted component of a radiographic image is called (a/n):

   a. artifact
   b. fog
   c. aliasing
   d. pixilation

6. If the technologist fails to detent the x-ray tube to the bucky or detector, which of the following is likely to occur?

   a. excessive patient dose
   b. excessive pixel brightness
   c. clipped anatomy of interest
   d. a nonexposed or blank image

7. Which of the following has/have no effect on spatial resolution?

   a. exposure index values
   b. motion
   c. monitor quality
   d. lp/mm

8. The greater the number of x-ray photons that strike the image receptor, the:

   a. greater the electronic noise
   b. better the penetration
   c. lower the patient dose
   d. higher the signal-to-noise ratio

9. If the central ray is placed so that it is not directed through the center of the anatomy, the radiographic image evaluation criteria most affected will be:

   a. image noise
   b. image contrast
   c. shape distortion
   d. spatial resolution

10. If the signal-to-noise ratio is less than optimal, what becomes more apparent on the image?

    a. Moiré effect
    b. shape distortion
    c. image graininess
    d. loss of contrast resolution

11. Image visualization is optimized when:

    a. pixel brightness is set to a scale of black and white
    b. penetration and kVp are minimal
    c. at least 8 LP/mm is resolved
    d. SNR settings are in the 100:1 to 200:1 range

12. If the sampling rate is the same as the line pairs resolution of the IP:

    a. spatial resolution reaches its peak
    b. scanning will occur twice
    c. aliasing artifacts may occur
    d. no image will result because the image signal and the electronic signal will cancel each other out

13. Which of the following situations could result in clipping anatomy in the superior or inferior portion of the IR?

    a. failing to detent
    b. not aligning the bucky tray with the central ray
    c. angling the central ray caudally
    d. increasing the field size

14. The source of electronic noise in a digital imaging system is:

    a. electrons
    b. scatter radiation
    c. the original signal
    d. inadequate exposure to the IR

15. Why is it important to remove IV lines and oxygen tubes from the exposure field?

    a. to ensure that image processing is not halted
    b. it keeps them from obscuring anatomy and/or pathology
    c. they create artificial brightness and gray scale on the image
    d. they can become entangled during scanning and injure the patient

For Questions 16 to 20, match the image evaluation criteria with its acceptable level of performance or the factors that affect it.

16. _____ Image contrast   a. Affected by focal spot size

17. _____ Artifacts   b. Occurs when OID is changed

18. _____ Spatial resolution c. No foreign objects should be visible

19. _____ Pixel brightness   d. Should be balanced with gray scale

20. _____ Size distortion   e. All pixel levels of gray should be visible

21. Moiré effect is more likely to occur when using which types of imaging equipment?

    1. CR reader
    2. Mobile x-ray unit
    3. Grids

    a. 1, 2
    b. 1, 3
    c. 2, 3
    d. 1, 2, 3

22. If graininess appears on an image, the most appropriate item to check in the list below is the:

    a. kVp setting
    b. image monitor
    c. bucky tray
    d. grid frequency

23. The recommended SNR for a CRT used for digital imaging is:

    a. 1:1
    b. 1:500
    c. 1,000:1
    d. 10:1

24. Moiré effect is more likely to occur when:

    a. the bucky tray is not pushed in completely
    b. the Nyquist frequency matches parallel grid lines
    c. no collimation is present
    d. the central ray is off from the IR in a superior direction

25. Which of the following does not have to be checked on an image to ensure that it is diagnostic?

    a. shape distortion
    b. adequate penetration
    c. CR reader used
    d. pixel brightness

Labeling

1. Evaluate the radiographs shown. Based on their appearance, identify the problem in each radiograph using the following choices: Moiré effect, removable artifacts present, and x-ray tube not detented.

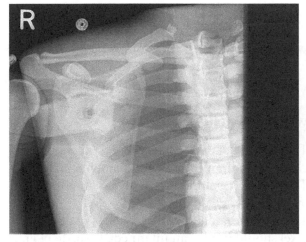 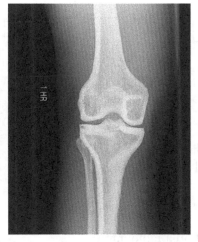 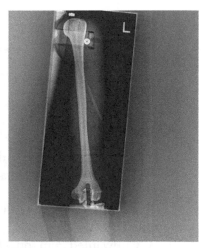

a) _____   b) _____   c) _____

Crossword Puzzle

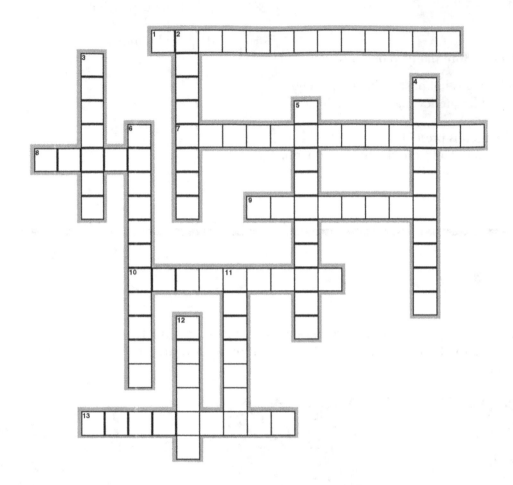

Across

1. A one-word term for size distortion
7. The preferred value digital fluoro for this type of ratio is 500:1 (hyphen)
8. This type of artifact is caused by grids; _____ effect
9. Any unwanted component on a radiograph
10. In order to avoid shape distortion or clipping anatomy, the technologist must ensure tube and bucky _____
13. An image may appear this way on a monitor when the image is so magnified that individual pixels can be seen

Down

2. Type of artifact due to the scanning frequency too closely aligning with the grid frequency
3. This type of resolution must be 8 lp/mm for optimum image quality
4. The image evaluation criteria that states that each pixel should display an intermediate shade of gray; pixel _____
5. The type of noise that is inherent in digital imaging systems due to the movement of electrons
6. Higher kVp settings ensures adequate _____; the ability of the x-ray beam to travel through the part
11. Refers to the sampling frequency of a CR reader; _____ frequency
12. This artifact becomes apparent if SNR's are too low

25

Digital Image Display

1. The type of display monitor that contains an electron gun and accelerating grids:

   a. primary
   b. secondary
   c. cathode ray tube
   d. liquid crystal diode

2. The environment inside a cathode ray tube would best be described as:

   a. nematic
   b. clean
   c. positively charged
   d. a vacuum

3. The anode side of a CRT:

   a. fluoresces when struck by electrons
   b. changes polarity after each horizontal trace
   c. is modulated using a TFT
   d. contains spherical glass spacers

4. When comparing viewing monitors, increased signal-to-noise ratios result in:

   a. larger field sizes
   b. sharper images
   c. degraded detail
   d. flicker

5. The configuration formed by a scanning electron gun in a CRT is termed a/n:

   a. raster pattern
   b. intensity modulation
   c. image matrix
   d. diagonal retrace

6. The focusing and accelerating grids in a cathode ray tube work on the electrical principle that:

   a. charge is greatest where the curvature is greatest
   b. like charges repel
   c. charge resides on the outside of a conductor
   d. distance affects the force of the attraction between two unlike charges

7. To ensure that flicker is not apparent when viewing radiographic images on a monitor:

   a. ambient light should be minimized or eliminated
   b. the signal-to-noise ratio must be at least 500:1
   c. the viewer must stand directly in front of the monitor
   d. the screen is refreshed every 33 ms

8. The deflection coil in an electron gun of a CRT serves to:

   a. accelerate the electrons
   b. aim the electrons at the cathode
   c. steer the electrons in a linear pattern
   d. pull the electrons outside the vacuum tube

9. If the electrical current is 60 Hz, _____ fields per second can be scanned using a cathode ray tube?

    a. 30
    b. 60
    c. 90
    d. 120

10. If the signal-to-noise ratio is less than optimal in a viewing device, what becomes more apparent on the image?

    a. veiling glare
    b. dead pixels
    c. image graininess
    d. flicker

11. The vertical resolution of a CRT is controlled by:

    a. the number of lines in the raster pattern
    b. the image's orientation (i.e., landscape vs. portrait)
    c. how many times the electron stream is modulated
    d. the magnitude of the video signal

12. If the bandpass of a viewing system is increased, the bit storage of the system will be:

    a. decreased
    b. increased also
    c. only increased if the frame rate decreases
    d. unaffected

13. How does frequency modulation in a viewing system affect spatial resolution?

    a. as frequency modulation increases, resolution decreases
    b. as frequency modulation increases, resolution increases
    c. as frequency modulation decreases, resolution increases
    d. no effect; frequency modulation does not affect resolution

14. In order to eliminate reflective glare when using an image viewing device, the technologist or radiologist should:

    a. increase the monitor brightness using the CRT's controls
    b. decrease the default window level
    c. view the image at 90 degrees, rather than from an angle
    d. lower the ambient light level

15. Veiling glare in a viewing system is commonly caused by:

    a. a SNR of less than 500:1
    b. the loss of signal at the periphery of the image
    c. light leakage and electron backscatter
    d. excessive scatter when imaging a large patient

16. Which of the following are advantages of a liquid crystal diode (LCD) over a conventional cathode ray tube (CRT)?

    1. Image is visible from multiple angles
    2. Lighter in weight
    3. Generates less heat

    a. 1, 2
    b. 1, 3
    c. 2, 3
    d. 1, 2, 3

17. Which of the following is true regarding liquid crystals used in LCD's?

    a. they generate a magnetic field to create the image
    b. the crystals only flow under high heat conditions
    c. each crystal is controlled by a spacer glass bead
    d. they are electrically charged

18. When a nematic liquid crystal is exposed to an external electric field, the crystals:

    a. flow more easily
    b. align
    c. reverse their polarity
    d. become electrically neutral

19. An LCD converts the image from an electrical signal by:

    a. using a gridded transparent conductor system in the panel
    b. placing an external magnetic field near the panel
    c. using an electron gun to create a line by line pattern
    d. increasing the signal-to-noise ratio by more than a thousand times

20. Compared to conventional computer monitors, medical viewing monitors must have higher:

    1. Brightness levels
    2. Signal-to-noise ratios
    3. Response times

    a. 1, 2
    b. 1,3
    c. 2, 3
    d. 1, 2, 3

21. An Active Matrix Liquid Crystal Display (AMLCD) creates an image:

    a. line by line
    b. column by column
    c. bead by bead
    d. pixel by pixel

22. The function in the thin-film transistor in an AMLCD is to:

    a. polarize the light emitted
    b. remove any excess charge in the bus lines
    c. maintain the integrity of the glass spacers
    d. maintain the brightness of each pixel

23. Both the LCD and AMLCD viewing devices contain:

    a. electron gun dipoles
    b. two glass plates encasing the active crystals
    c. a phosphor layer
    d. deflection coils

24. For medical imaging, it is recommended that an active matrix liquid crystal display device be:

    a. equipped with a backscatter grid
    b. have red, green, or blue filters in each pixel
    c. monochromatic
    d. set at a frame rate of 60 frame/s or higher

25. One measure of AMLCD performance is response time. Response time is best described as:

    a. the time it takes for the phosphor to fluoresce
    b. the time needed for pixel brightness to change
    c. the time required to recharge the detector array
    d. the time interval before the next frame can be reconstructed

26. The LCD or AMLCD able to provide the highest resolution image would have:

    a. a matrix size in the megapixel range
    b. fewer frequency modulations
    c. increased light energy scatter
    d. decreased backlight emission

27. Which of the following are disadvantages of LCD and AMLCD display systems?

    1. They come in only flat screens
    2. Finger pressure on the screen can cause permanent damage
    3. Optimal viewing occurs at a 90-degree angle

    a. 1, 2
    b. 1, 3
    c. 2, 3
    d. 1, 2, 3

28. The class of display workstations required to be used for the interpretation of medical images is called:

    a. primary
    b. dipole
    c. substrate
    d. secondary

29. According to AAPM Task Group 18 requirements, luminance levels of image display monitors should be at least:

    a. 8 bits/trace
    b. 480 × 640
    c. 171 candelas/m^2
    d. set so that no reflective glare is present

30. After viewing an image and adjusting the window level and window width to more optimal levels, the technologist should:

    a. save the changes and send the image to PACS for interpretation
    b. first restore the image to its initial appearance, save it, and then send it for interpretation
    c. select a larger field of view in proportion to the changes and then send for interpretation
    d. not save any changes and send for interpretation

Labeling

1. Label the components of a cathode ray tube (CRT).

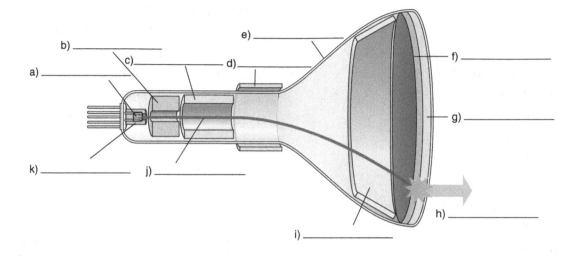

2. Identify the following items in the diagrams illustrating the formation of a complete television field by filling in the blanks provided: the horizontal retrace and the vertical retrace in the first frame, the missing numerals of the retrace lines in the second frame, and the total number of lines that make up the final television field in the third frame.

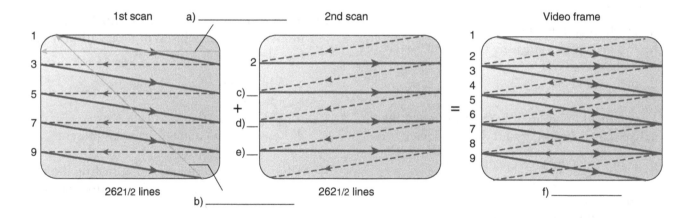

3. Label the components that make up one pixel in an active matrix liquid crystal display (AMLCD).

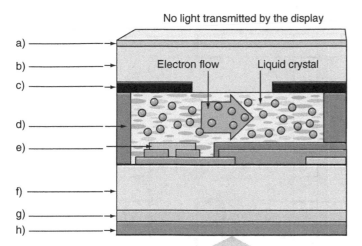
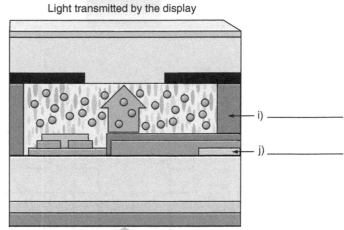

Crossword Puzzle

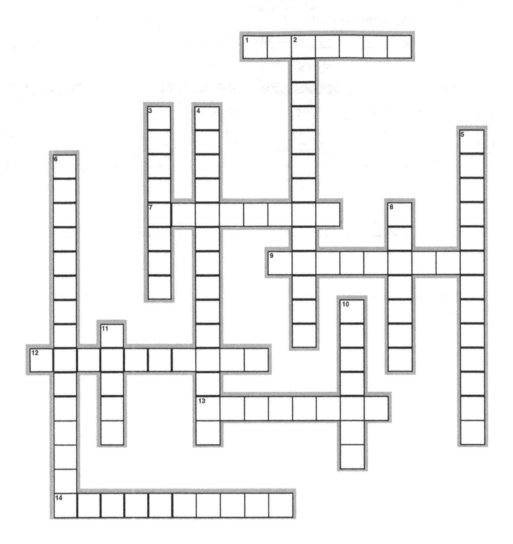

Across

1. Term used to describe the electrically-charged and linear-shaped crystal molecules used in LCDs
7. The portion of the CRT that fluoresces when struck by a stream of electrons
9. Device in AMLCD that prevents charge from leaking out of the liquid crystal cells
12. The type of trace in a raster pattern scan when the electron beam returns to the original corner of the scan but continues the pattern on the third line until all the odd-numbered lines are completed
13. The conductors used in AMLCD that controls each pixel with a TFT (two words)
14. Can occur when too much pressure is applied to the monitor when pointing out anatomy; damage to the monitor that cannot be repaired (two words)

Down

2. Type of AMLCD monitor used to display medical images, allowing images to be displayed in shades from white to black
3. Another term for frequency modulations
4. Conventional television device (three words)
5. Created by the electron gun as it scans across the phosphor screen line by line (two words)
6. Each scan from the top to the bottom of a screen is called a _____ _____ (two words)
8. Type of glare that results due to the internal workings of the CRT monitor
10. Time required to reconstruct the next frame in an LCD: _____ time
11. The distance from the middle of one pixel to the middle of the next pixel is called pixel _____.

26

Digital Image Management

1. An advantage of PACS is that it allows images to be:

   a. stored in hard copy format
   b. saved to prevent image manipulation after exposure
   c. sent to several workstations and monitors simultaneously
   d. created using film and automatic processing

2. Data compression:

   a. results in faster processing
   b. produces faster transmission times
   c. requires less storage space
   d. does all of the above

3. The set of computer standards used to permit a wide range of digital imaging systems to ensure that images taken at one facility are able to viewed correctly at another facility is termed:

   a. DICOM
   b. PACS
   c. PSP
   d. TFT

4. In order to preserve spatial resolution, the preferred compression method is:

   a. lossy
   b. lossless
   c. RAID-based
   d. interfaced with an SSL

5. What role does a RAID play in a PACS network?

   a. it ensures there are no bugs in the system
   b. it acts as a security layer
   c. it allows all users to interface with it using barcode readers
   d. it ensures there is sufficient memory in the system and prevents image loss

6. The function of the image manager and server in a PACS system is to:

   a. digitize analog film images
   b. create redundant soft copies of an image
   c. allow the PACS to interface with the HIS
   d. act as a database for directing images to all the network's devices

7. What advantage does routing by the image manager in a PACS system provide to a medical imaging department?

   a. it automatically filters exams by type so that each imaging area only views and receives that day's relevant worklist
   b. it compresses images to JPEG formats for faster image transmission
   c. it ensures that HL7 standards are met by all devices in the network
   d. it prevents wrong patient information to be entered into the system

8. **Which of the following is NOT a function or responsibility of a HIS?**

    a. responsible for transmitting patient EMR's using HL7 standards
    b. must be compatible with PACS and RIS
    c. troubleshoots and calibrates image monitors
    d. provides access to lab tests, medical images, and physician notes

9. **What undesirable result would occur if a patient's name is not consistent throughout the PACS system?**

    1. Lost images
    2. Data breaches
    3. Missed diagnoses

    a. 1, 2
    b. 1, 3
    c. 2, 3
    d. 1, 2, 3

10. **The two types of image acquisition modalities in a PACS network are:**

    a. frame grabbers and those that are fundamentally digital
    b. lossy and lossless
    c. LCD-based and CRT-based
    d. HIS and RIS

For Questions 11 to 15, match the term or acronym with its appropriate definition or description.

11. _____ LAN
12. _____ Worklist
13. _____ HL7
14. _____ ACR
15. _____ RIS

    a. Professional society for radiologists
    b. Small network of devices; geographically limited
    c. Generated by the image manager; exam orders for day
    d. Network for medical images, billing, and reports
    e. Communication standard for all EMR's

16. **For interpretation purposes, the workstation used by the radiologist should be at least _____ for image viewing.**

    a. 1,024 pixels
    b. 1 megapixels
    c. 2 megapixels
    d. 10 kilopixels

17. **The compression ratio below that is the most likely to allow an image to still be diagnostic after compressing and sending it through PACS is:**

    a. 2:1
    b. 10:1
    c. 50:1
    d. 100:1

18. **If it is found that a network device is not DICOM-compatible, this would mostly likely result in:**

    a. artifacts on the image
    b. network malfunctions
    c. excessive file sizes
    d. HL7 compliance

19. **The preferred workstation viewing device of those listed below is a/n:**

    a. CRT
    b. TCP/IP
    c. MOD
    d. LCD

20. **A device that could be used for long-term archiving of medical images is a/n:**

    a. DB file
    b. jukebox
    c. hard copy
    d. frame grabber

21. **What information could be found in the DICOM header of an image?**

    1. Patient name
    2. Date of procedure
    3. Position of patient

    a. 1, 2
    b. 1, 3
    c. 2, 3
    d. 1, 2, 3

22. **The DICOM standards were developed by which two professional organizations?**

    a. ARRT and ASRT
    b. EMR and HIPAA
    c. RIS and CCD
    d. ACR and NEMA

23. If a facility initially only sets up a mini-PACS this means that:

    a. the network may be limited to only one modality
    b. the workstations are designed for shorter technologists
    c. the workstations are mobile, allowing greater department flexibility
    d. the network will have no archival ability

24. When would a technologist typically query the archive using the image manager?

    a. to initiate the image compression process
    b. to locate the patient and verify his/her identifiers
    c. to check the latest HL7 standards in the United States
    d. to retrieve any previous exams

25. The patient's full EMR would most likely be found in the:

    a. ACR
    b. PACS
    c. HIS
    d. TCP/IP

For Questions 26 to 30, determine if each statement is true or false. Use a) for true and b) for false.

26. _____ It is best to annotate the right or left side after exposure.

27. _____ An image saved in a JPEG (Joint Photography Experts) format would meet lossless compression standards.

28. _____ It would be appropriate for a QC technologist to use a higher resolution monitor while performing his/her duties.

29. _____ A DICOM-compliant device ensures patient confidentiality.

30. _____ The DICOM Presentation State standard outlines the requirements for capturing and storing any adjustments made to the image after exposure.

Labeling

1. Identify and label each component of this mini-PACS network: the storage server, the network interface, and the display monitor.

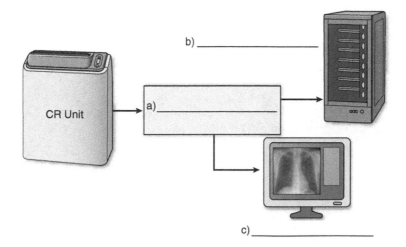

CR Unit

a) _____

b) _____

c) _____

2. **Evaluate the radiographs to determine which type of compression, lossy (irreversible) or loss-less (reversible), was used to send and display each image. Place your answers in the boxes provided.**

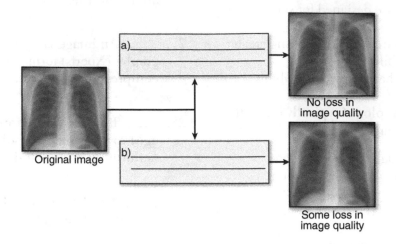

Crossword Puzzle

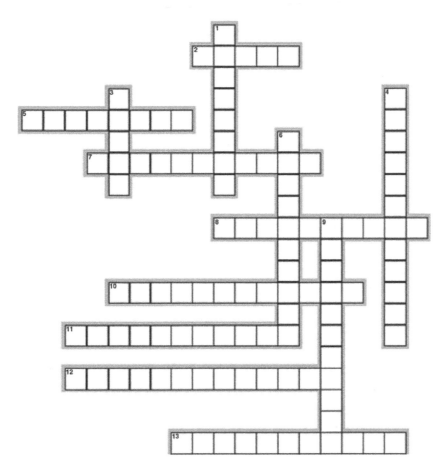

Across

2. Type of compression that is irreversible in terms of image quality
5. The portion of PACS responsible for storing the images (plural)
7. Process of reducing an image's file size
8. The radiologist's monitor must meet this standard of 2 _____.
10. The types of digital image acquisition device that digitizes analog signals received from the IR (two words)
11. Each vendor and modality highlights how well their device meets the DICOM _____ statement
12. The patient's entire health documentation in network-ready format; electronic _____ _____ (two words)
13. The network that functions within the medical imaging department; encompasses PACS, reports, and billing; radiology _____ system

Down

1. The schedule of patients and the exams they are due to have; generated by the image manager
3. Digital imaging and communications in medicine
4. General name for a type of long-term image that includes MOD's and DVD's (two words)
6. The ability of each vendor's devices to interface with each other in the network; DICOM-_____
9. A device used for short- and long-term storage; redundant array of _____ disks

PART V

Specialized Imaging Techniques

Fluoroscopy

27

1. The input phosphor of an image intensifier is coated with _____ and the output phosphor is made of _____:

   a. zinc cadmium sulfide (ZnCdS); cesium iodide (Csl)
   b. calcium tungstate (CaWO$_4$); zinc cadmium sulfide (ZnCdS)
   c. cesium iodide (Csl); zinc cadmium sulfide (ZnCdS)
   d. cesium iodide (Csl); calcium tungstate (CaWO$_4$)

2. The output phosphor of an image intensifier converts:

   a. electron energy into light photons
   b. light photons into electrons
   c. light photons into x-rays
   d. electrons into x-rays

3. The electrostatic lenses of an image intensifier:

   a. convert electron energy into light photons
   b. convert x-ray energy into light photons
   c. convert light photons into electrons
   d. focus electrons to converge on the output phosphor

4. The primary disadvantage of using the magnification mode rather than the standard image mode on an image intensifier is that it:

   a. increases image magnification
   b. increases the patient dose
   c. produces a higher-resolution image
   d. produces a brighter image

5. In an image intensifier tube, the _____ gain occurs because the input diameter is larger than the output diameter:

   a. minification
   b. confiscation
   c. flux
   d. radiation

6. _____ gain is due to the acceleration of the photoelectrons:

   a. Magnification
   b. Confiscation
   c. Flux
   d. Radiation

7. Flux gain and minification gain can be multiplied together to determine:

   a. image magnification
   b. total image resolution
   c. total brightness gain
   d. automatic brightness control

8. The ABC circuit automatically adjusts the:

   a. conversion of brightness to electrons
   b. input brightness of the image intensifier tube
   c. output brightness of the image intensifier tube
   d. brightness of the ambient light available

9. The ABC circuit adjusts _____ to maintain _____.

   a. constant brightness; constant mA or kVp
   b. mA or kVp; constant brightness
   c. mA or kVp; constant patient thickness
   d. patient thickness; constant brightness

10. The _____ in the eye are used for viewing in dim light.

   a. rods
   b. cones
   c. optic disc
   d. olfactory bulb

11. Image intensification is consistently used as an accessory device for fluoroscopy. Its primary purpose is to:

   a. allow more than one person to view the image at one time
   b. increase the brightness levels of the original image
   c. reduce patient skin dose
   d. shorten overall exam time

12. Fluoroscopic mA currents are in the range from:

   a. 0.5 to 5 mA
   b. 50 to 100 mA
   c. 100 to 200 mA
   d. 300 to 400 mA

13. The minimum distance between the source and the patient's skin surface (SSD) for a fixed fluoroscopic unit is _____ cm.

   a. 15
   b. 30
   c. 38
   d. 42

14. The fluoroscopic timer must have an audible signal which is heard when _____ minutes of fluoroscopy time have elapsed.

   a. 2
   b. 5
   c. 10
   d. 15

15. Fluoroscopy is utilized to observe moving structures in the body. This is termed:

   a. static imaging
   b. dynamic imaging
   c. magnification imaging
   d. spot film imaging

16. When digital fluoroscopy is used, which of the following devices replace devices used in conventional fluoroscopy?

   1. CCD
   2. ABS
   3. DFPD

   a. 1, 2
   b. 1, 3
   c. 2, 3
   d. 1, 2, 3

17. When the output image is digitized and continuously displayed on the fluoroscopy monitor, this is known as:

   a. last image hold
   b. magnification
   c. automatic brightness control
   d. brightness gain

18. Which of the following devices is responsible for converting the light image from the output phosphor into an electric signal?

   a. beam-splitting mirror
   b. input phosphor
   c. cathode ray tube (CRT)
   d. video camera tube

19. The ICRU recommends that the following formula be used to evaluate the performance of an image intensifier's brightness production:

   a. I^2/O^2
   b. flux gain X minification gain
   c. # output light photons/# of input x-ray photons
   d. output phosphor luminance/input phosphor luminance

20. An intensifier has a flux gain of 45 and a minification gain of 230. Determine the total brightness gain for this unit.

    a. 26
    b. 275
    c. 2,025
    d. 10,350

21. An image intensifier has the following dimensions: Input phosphor = 12 cm. Output phosphor = 3.5 cm. Compute and select the minification gain below:

    a. 15.5
    b. 11.8
    c. 8.5
    d. 3.4

22. A particular image intensifier tube has a flux gain of 75. The diameter of the input phosphor is 15 cm and the diameter of the output phosphor is 3 cm. The total gain for this image intensifier tube is about:

    a. 375
    b. 1,125
    c. 1,875
    d. 18,750

23. What is the device that directs the light emitted from the image intensifier to various viewing and imaging apparatus?

    a. spot film changer
    b. output phosphor
    c. beam splitter
    d. automatic brightness control

24. The input phosphor of an image intensifier is responsible for converting:

    a. x-rays to light
    b. x-rays to electrons
    c. light to electrons
    d. electrons to light

25. Which of the following factors would affect quantum mottle the most?

    a. OID
    b. focal point position
    c. minification geometry
    d. tube mA

26. Federal requirements limit total fluoroscopy tube output to:

    a. 5,000 mrems/year
    b. 10 R/minute
    c. 100 mR/hour
    d. 1 R/day at 1 m

27. Reduced image brightness on the periphery of a fluoroscopy image due to the concave shape of the input phosphor is called:

    a. vignetting
    b. variations
    c. zooming
    d. mottling

28. The fluoroscopy device that uses cesium iodide and amorphous silicon to produce a dynamic image is a/n:

    a. image intensifier
    b. input phosphor
    c. indirect capture flat panel
    d. charge-coupled device

29. Which of the following are advantages of charged-coupled devices over video camera tubes?

    1. Little to no lag
    2. High DQE
    3. Increased spatial resolution

    a. 1, 2
    b. 1,3
    c. 2, 3
    d. 1, 2, 3

30. Select the items that would serve to increase patient dose during fluoroscopy?

    1. Increasing SSD
    2. Using magnification mode
    3. Increasing SID during mobile fluoroscopy

    a. 1, 2
    b. 1, 3
    c. 2, 3
    d. 1, 2, 3

Labeling

1. Label the components of a modern radiographic and fluoroscopic (R & F) room.

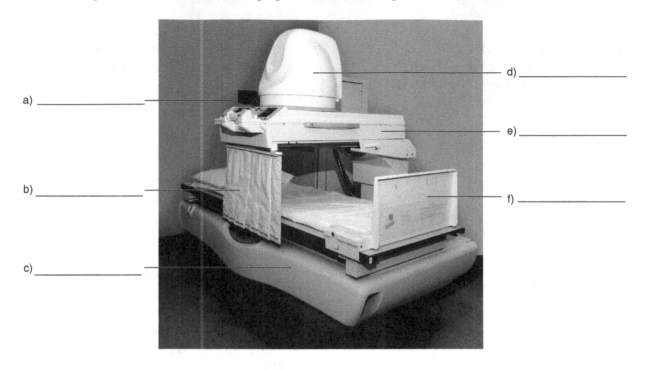

a) _____

b) _____

c) _____

d) _____

e) _____

f) _____

2. Identify the lettered components of the image intensifier tube.

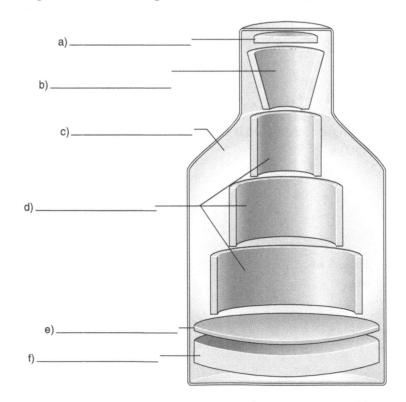

a) _____

b) _____

c) _____

d) _____

e) _____

f) _____

3. Label components a to j for the video camera tube shown.

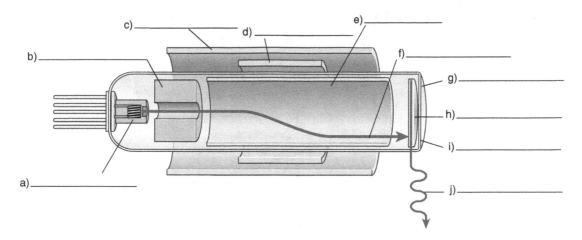

Crossword Puzzle:

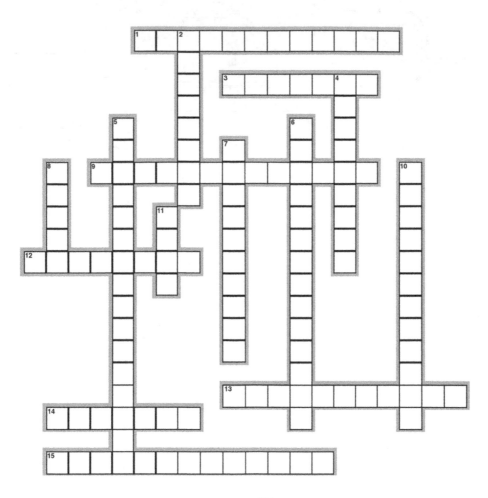

Across

1. Phosphor used in the input phosphor of an I.I. and in an indirect capture flat panel device
3. Unit for luminance; used in the calculation of an image intensifier's conversion factor
9. Fluoroscopic operating mode where the object is made to appear larger than its actual size
12. The semiconducting material used in a fluoroscopic direct capture flat panel device; amorphous _____
13. Term for the technique used to produce a real time, dynamic imaging study using x-rays
14. The most common type of video camera tube used in fluoroscopy TV systems
15. The device that replaces a video camera tube when digital fluoroscopy is used (hyphenated)

Down

2. Type of vision used in dim light; controlled by the rods in the eye
4. The material used for the target plate in a plumbicon video camera tube (two words)
5. Device that converts x-rays to light, making the image up to 8,000 times brighter (two words)
6. Component of the image intensifier that converts electrons to light (two words)
7. Occurs at the edges of a fluoroscopic image due to the concave curve of the output phosphor
8. Fluoroscopic operating mode where the x-ray generators are synchronized to generate x-rays only when the camera shutter is open
10. Type of brightness gain that occurs in an I.I. due to the differences in input and output phosphor diameters
11. Type of brightness gain that occurs in an I.I. due to the acceleration of electrons

Imaging Equipment

28

1. During linear tomography, which of the following motions are synchronized to move in opposite directions?

   a. x-ray tube and image receptor
   b. x-ray tube anode and cathode
   c. image receptor and the object
   d. image receptor and the bucky

2. The larger the tomographic angle, the:

   a. thicker the cut or object plane
   b. thinner the cut or object plane
   c. faster the cut
   d. larger the body part

3. The advantage of tomography is improved:

   a. density
   b. ability to see superimposed structures
   c. detail
   d. patient exposure

4. The location of the object plane is determined by the:

   a. focal spot size
   b. tomographic angle
   c. SID
   d. fulcrum location

5. When performing linear tomography, the most appropriate technical factors to select would be:

   a. increased time and low mA
   b. decreased time and low mA
   c. increased time and high mA
   d. decreased time and high mA

6. Which of the following are true regarding exposure arc?

   1. It is always longer than tomographic arc
   2. It represents the time that x-rays are emitted from the tube
   3. It plays a role in determining object plane thickness

   a. 1, 2
   b. 1, 3
   c. 2, 3
   d. 1, 2, 3

7. With regard to linear tomography, the anatomy that is the greatest distance from the fulcrum or focal plane will be:

   a. the most sharply imaged
   b. subject to ghosting
   c. the most blurred
   d. resuperimposed

8. When performing an IV urogram (IVU), the most appropriate section thickness would be:

   a. 5 mm
   b. 2 mm
   c. 3 cm
   d. 1 cm

9. If a 6-degree tomographic angle is used, the approximate thickness of the focal plane will be:

   a. 31 mm
   b. 16 mm
   c. 11 mm
   d. 3 mm

10. The tomographic movement that would be able to image the smallest anatomic structures would most likely be:

    a. linear
    b. circular
    c. elliptical
    d. hypocycloidal

For Questions 11 to 15, place the steps of performing a tomographic exposure in the correct order by matching each step with its appropriate description:

11. _____ Step 1   a. The tube and IR move synchronously during exposure

12. _____ Step 2   b. The x-ray exposure starts and x-rays are emitted

13. _____ Step 3   c. Tube movement ends

14. _____ Step 4   d. The tube and IR are returned to their starting positions

15. _____ Step 5   e. Tube movement begins

16. The type of tomography performed where the tube and IR move synchronously around a patient's head is:

    a. panoramic tomography
    b. computed tomography
    c. linear tomography
    d. positron emission tomography

17. The anatomy best demonstrated using a dedicated panorex unit is/are the:

    a. orbits and cervical spine
    b. facial bones and auricles
    c. gonion, acanthion, and inion
    d. mandible

18. The advantages of using a dedicated chest unit are:

    a. increased department efficiency and patient throughput
    b. greater ability to set individualized exposure factors
    c. variable SIDs
    d. fewer positioning or infection control concerns

19. Mobile radiography could be used in which of the following medical settings?

    1. Surgery
    2. Intensive care unit
    3. Emergency department

    a. 1, 2
    b. 1, 3
    c. 2, 3
    d. 1, 2, 3

20. If a technologist takes a capacitor discharge mobile radiographic unit and attempts to perform several bedside portable chest exposures without plugging the unit into an outlet each time, which of the following is likely to occur?

    a. the unit will not be able to expose the IR
    b. the first few chest exposures will be fine, but exposures may not be present on the last exams
    c. nothing; this type of unit does not need to be plugged in for exposures
    d. the unit cannot be transported unless it is plugged in

21. Which of the radiographic image qualities will be affected the most if the correct SID is not used during mobile radiography?

    a. contrast
    b. magnification
    c. brightness
    d. noise

22. If a radiographer is not able to obtain the full 72″ required for a portable AP chest x-ray ordered on a semiconscious ICU patient, she/he should:

    a. use a 40″ rib technique from one of the department's units
    b. use the 72″ AP chest technique she/he usually uses and use postprocessing to visualize the anatomy
    c. measure and annotate the actual SID used and adjust mAs downward
    d. transport the patient to the department using a cart and the full 72″

23. Grid cutoff during a mobile radiographic exam is more likely to occur:

   a. if the tube and IR are not aligned side to side
   b. when using lower ratio grids
   c. during small extremity exposures
   d. if the patient moves during the exposure

24. For radiation protection purposes during a mobile radiographic exposure, the radiographer should:

   a. wear a lead apron during the exposure
   b. place himself/herself at least 6 feet away from the patient
   c. stand at a 90-degree angle to the patient
   d. complete all of these actions

25. What undesirable effect will occur if a radiographer fails to properly set the equipment locks while transporting the portable unit or performing mobile radiography?

   a. the patient's anatomy may appear foreshortened
   b. line fluctuations will cause the unit's technical factors to be off
   c. the x-ray tube could become broken or damaged
   d. the ability to make exposures will automatically be disabled

Labeling

1. Identify each of the following tomographic exposure components shown in the diagram: fulcrum, tomographic angle, object plane, and exposure angle.

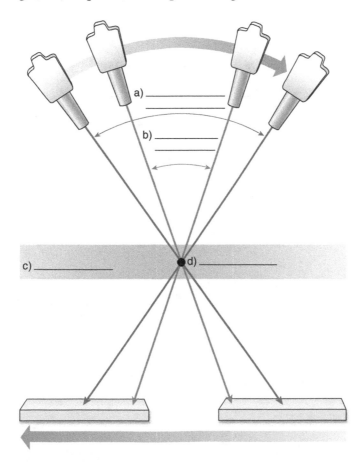

2. Evaluate the two tomographic exposure diagrams. Based on their appearance and the resulting slice thicknesses of each, label the exposure obtained at 30 degrees and the exposure obtained at 60 degrees.

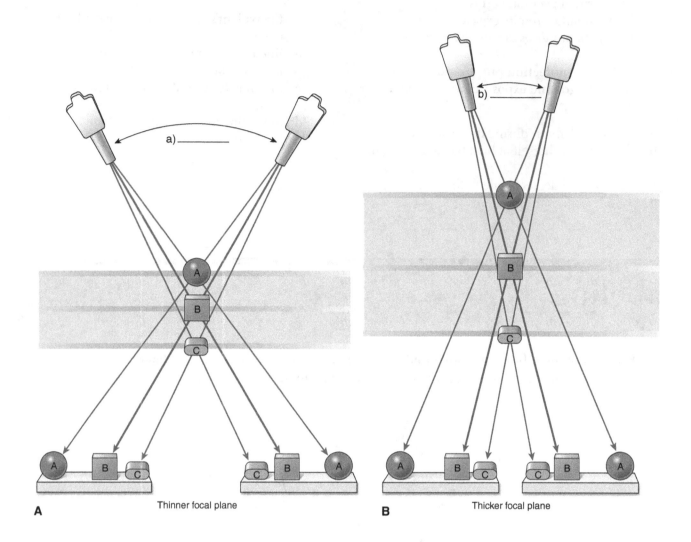

a) _____

b) _____

A   Thinner focal plane

B   Thicker focal plane

Crossword Puzzle

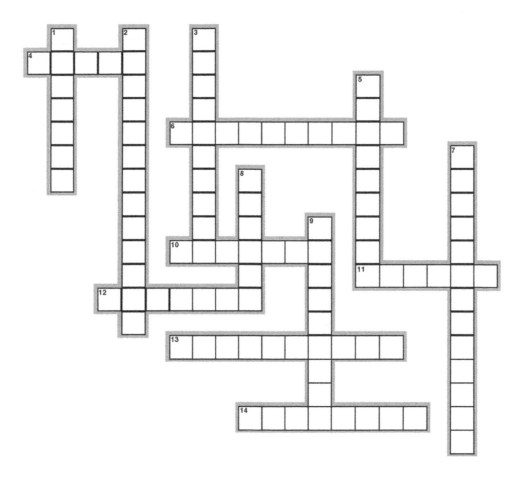

Across

4. This piece of equipment is electronically connected to the x-ray tube in a dedicated chest unit, allowing both to move up and down synchronously
6. The level of anatomy most sharply imaged during tomography (two words)
10. The relationship between tomographic arc and section thickness
11. The undesirable result if a radiographer uses too high of a grid ratio or uses a grid improperly during portable exams; grid _____ (hyphenated)
12. A type of mobile fluoroscopic unit that does not need an outlet to take an exposure but does need to be recharged
13. Special imaging technique that blurs out anatomy outside the plane of interest using tube motion
14. The anatomy best demonstrated when using a panorex dedicated x-ray unit

Down

1. Determines the level of the object plane in linear tomography
2. One of the most complex motions in tomography; allows small anatomic structures to be visualized
3. The radiographic quality most affected if the x-ray tube and IR are not level with each other during a mobile radiographic exposure
5. Type of tomography that is completed by having the tube and the IR move around the patient's head
7. This radiographic quality will be undesirably increased during mobile radiography if the routine SID is not used
8. The angle (number of degrees) a radiographer should stand with regard to the patient during portable radiographic exams for radiation protection purposes
9. Term used to denote x-ray units that are used for very specific exams only

Quality Assurance and Control

29

1. The sum of the difference between the light and the x-ray field edges must be within ___ of the SID.

   a. 1%
   b. 2%
   c. 5%
   d. 10%

2. The _____ can be used to measure digital imaging display monitor quality.

   a. pinhole camera
   b. SMPTE pattern
   c. step wedge
   d. sensitometer

3. The _____ measures the size of the focal spot.

   a. pinhole camera
   b. optical densitometer
   c. spinning top
   d. bar phantom

4. The kVp of the beam should be within (+/−) _____ % of the kVp setting.

   a. 2
   b. 5
   c. 7
   d. 10

5. The penetrability or filtration of an x-ray beam is reported in terms of its:

   a. EMG
   b. RTV
   c. HVL
   d. MAQ

6. The same mAs values achieved with several different mA and time settings must produce the same radiation output within _____ % of the average.

   a. +/−2
   b. +/−5
   c. +/−10
   d. +/−20

7. A quality control program includes:

   1. Periodic testing of equipment
   2. Acceptance testing
   3. Correcting deviations from expected equipment performance

   a. 1, 2
   b. 1, 3
   c. 2, 3
   d. 1, 2, 3

8. During the exposure linearity test, the mR/mAs should vary by no more than + or – % from the average.

    a. 2
    b. 5
    c. 7
    d. 10

9. In this series of four different exposures, which mA station does not meet the exposure linearity criteria?

    a. 50 mA, 3.2 mR/mAs
    b. 100 mAs, 5.8 mR/mAs
    c. 200 mAs, 6.0 mR/mAs
    d. 400 mAs, 6.2 mR/mAs

10. The test that would NOT be conducted as part of AEC quality control is:

    a. ion chamber sensitivity
    b. backup timer verification
    c. exposure reproducibility
    d. field uniformity

11. According to the data below, would the radiographic unit being tested meet the federal guidelines for reproducibility? Exposure #1 has a machine output (mR) of 246, #2 is 210, #3 is 239, #4 is 259, and #5 is 250.

    a. yes, it is within the accuracy guidelines
    b. no, it is outside the accuracy guidelines
    c. not enough information to tell the accuracy guidelines
    d. reproducibility is not a standard QC test for mA stations

12. For optimum radiation protection, lead aprons and thyroid shields should be checked:

    a. semiannually, using a resolution test tool
    b. annually, visually and radiographically
    c. annually, using a water phantom
    d. semiannually, placing the apron over an R-meter

13. Which of the following processor maintenance activities should be conducted daily?

    a. clean and rinse the deep tanks and racks
    b. take out and rinse crossover racks
    c. inspect all belts, pulleys, and gears for proper operation
    d. verify the replenishment rate

14. A radiograph comes out of the processor with numerous dark, tree-like markings. These most likely are caused by:

    a. acute bending of the film
    b. static electricity
    c. the safelight
    d. water on the loading bench

15. Any unwanted component of a radiographic image is called a(n):

    a. artifact
    b. fog
    c. plus (+) density
    d. minus (−) density

16. An artifact caused by the automatic processor is:

    a. static
    b. crease marks
    c. pi marks
    d. double exposure

17. Which of the following would be classified as an exposure artifact, occurring in film/screen or digital environments?

    a. guideshoe marks
    b. static
    c. dead pixels
    d. patient jewelry

18. Which of the following artifacts is the most likely to result if a computed radiography imaging plate was incompletely erased?

    a. phantom or ghost images
    b. negative densities
    c. dichroic staining
    d. light spots

19. The maximum exposure rate for a fluoroscopic unit is:

    a. + or −5% of the first day tested
    b. 10 R/min
    c. 5 R/y
    d. + or −10% of the highest mA setting

20. If the x-ray field is smaller than that indicated by the indicator knob on the collimator, a technologist risks:

    a. excessive patient exposure
    b. excessive density on the radiograph
    c. cutting off anatomy of interest
    d. a nonexposed (or blank) film

21. Quality control standards require that the exposure time must be _____ from what is set.

    a. + or −5%
    b. + or −10%
    c. + or −2%
    d. + or −10 ms

22. Which of the following tools would be appropriate to conduct a filtration or HVL QC test?

    a. pinhole camera
    b. spinning top
    c. aluminum sheets
    d. metallic markers

23. If a computed radiography imaging phosphor becomes cracked or scratched, leaving minus density artifacts on the radiograph, which of the following actions should be taken to solve this problem?

    a. use the window and level functions to correct the minus densities
    b. clean the phosphor using only the appropriate solution
    c. re-erase the plate in the laser reader
    d. replace the entire phosphor in the imaging plate

24. Which of the following organizations provide protocols and/or recommendations for digital imaging quality control?

    1. ACR
    2. AAPM
    3. NCRP

    a. 1, 2
    b. 1, 3
    c. 2, 3
    d. 1, 2, 3

25. If a technologist notices that there are white dots on a black background on the display monitor, the likely problem is:

    a. inadequate luminance
    b. excessive noise
    c. dead pixels
    d. quantum mottle

26. A photometer would be used to conduct which of the following digital imaging QC tests?

    a. erasure thoroughness
    b. monitor luminance
    c. spatial resolution
    d. gray scale

27. Which of the following monitor tests would require the workstation to be turned off?

    a. voltage fluctuation testing
    b. stuck pixels
    c. monitor luminance
    d. screen reflectance

28. In general, when and/or how often should digital QC tests be conducted to ensure diagnostic images?

    a. annually
    b. upon installation and at regular intervals thereafter
    c. acceptance testing is all that is required
    d. daily or whenever there is a problem

29. The ACR and AAPM recommend that display resolution be at least:

    a. 1.0 Lp/mm
    b. 2.5 Lp/mm
    c. 5.0 Lp/mm
    d. 10.0 Lp/mm

30. Protective apparel should be inspected _____ using _____.

    a. annually; fluoroscopy
    b. daily; a magnifying glass
    c. semiannually; an AAPM pattern
    d. monthly; a dosimeter

Labeling

1. Complete the table identifying the frequency, acceptance limits, and the test tool required for each equipment quality control test.

Factor	Monitoring Frequency	Limits	Test Tool
1. Focal spot size spatial resolution			
2. Collimation			
3. kVp			
4. Filtration/HVL			
5. Exposure time			
6. Exposure reproducibility			
7. Exposure linearity			
8. AEC			

2. Evaluate the radiographs and identify the type of artifact density illustrated (plus or minus). For each radiograph, also determine the category(ies) of each artifact based on its cause. NOTE: Some figures may have more than one type of artifact.

a) Type of artifact density: _____

b) Artifact category(ies): _____

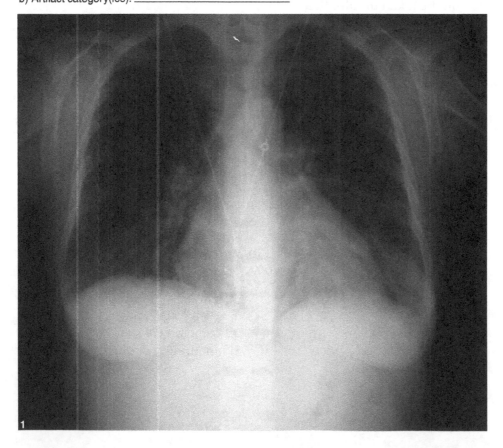

a) Type of artifact density: _____

b) Artifact category(ies): _____

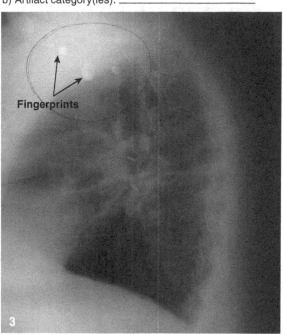

a) Type of artifact density: _____

b) Artifact category(ies): _____

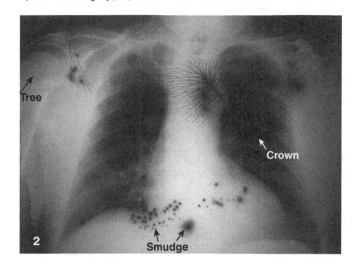

a) Type of artifact density: _____

b) Artifact category(ies): _____

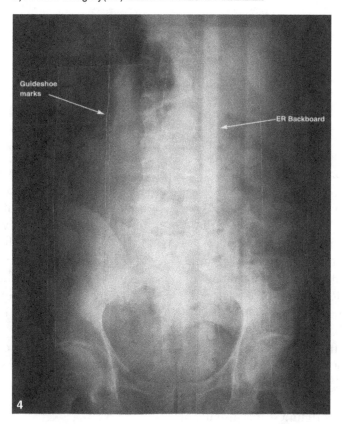

Crossword Puzzle

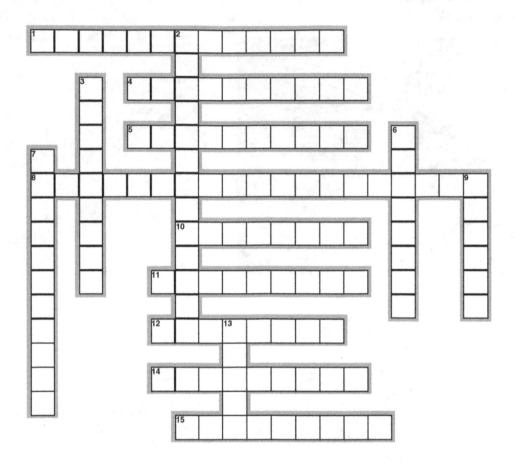

Across

1. This group has originated a pattern often used to check the brightness, contrast, and resolution of a display monitor: Society of _____ _____ and Television Engineers (two words)
4. This term describes the proper alignment of the light field and the x-ray field
5. QC tool used to check monitor display luminance
8. QC test that ensures that no ghost or residual image remains on the IR (two words)
10. Any unwanted information on a radiograph
11. A white dot on a black background visible on a display monitor screen; indicates a nonfunctional part of the display (two words)
12. Examples of this class of artifacts include crease marks, static, and light leaks
14. This measure of monitor brightness may use lux or candelas/m² as its unit of value
15. Individual the most qualified to run the more intensive and invasive digital imaging QC tests

Down

2. QC test tool used to check for the accuracy of the focal spot size (two words)
3. The QC test used to indicate that each mA station's output is within 10% of each other
6. The frequency interval that protective apparel should be checked for integrity
7. This monitor test is completed to ensure that the user cannot see his/her clothing or furniture on a monitor that has been turned off
9. Type of artifact due to inadequate levels of humidity
13. The frequency that each crossover rack in an automatic processor should be removed and rinsed

Computed Tomography

30

1. **An x-ray tube in a CT scanner has:**

   a. two cathodes
   b. a high heat capacity
   c. a molybdenum anode
   d. a stationary anode

2. **Indexing refers to the:**

   a. amount of table movement
   b. tube rotation speed
   c. rotations per centimeter of patient motion
   d. changes in high voltage

3. **A voxel is:**

   a. a picture element
   b. a volume element
   c. a data storage element
   d. the pixels arranged in columns and rows

4. **Detectors used in CT scanners are:**

   1. Solid state
   2. Vacuum tubes
   3. Scintillation based

   a. 1, 2
   b. 1, 3
   c. 2, 3
   d. 1, 2, 3

5. **The crystal of choice in current CT scintillation detectors is:**

   a. sodium iodide
   b. xenon
   c. cadmium tungstate
   d. carbon graphite

6. **The patient support table:**

   a. is made of low attenuation material
   b. is portable and may be used for patient transport
   c. has no relationship to the pitch
   d. contains the detector elements

7. **Spatial resolution describes the _____ of two objects that can be distinguished as separate objects.**

   a. Hounsfield unit
   b. minimum separation
   c. maximum size
   d. absorption differential

8. **Contrast resolution describes the ability to distinguish the _____ of two objects.**

   a. separation
   b. attenuation difference
   c. motion
   d. size

9. **Maximum intensity projection (MIP) is best described as:**

   a. a quality control test used to measure the maximum brightness of pixels
   b. a technique used to minimize the effect of streak artifacts
   c. a 3D multiplanar technique used to reconstruct CTA examinations
   d. one of the routine image reconstructions used for all CT exams

10. **The computer programs or formulae that calculate the CT numbers are called:**

    a. Pym programs
    b. shaded contrast diagrams
    c. Hounsfield units
    d. algorithms

11. **The CT number of fat is:**

    a. −1,000
    b −100
    c. 0
    d. 1,000

12. **The CT number for bone is closest to:**

    a. −1,000
    b. −50
    c. 0
    d. +1,000

13. **Reverse display can be used to:**

    a. convert a hard copy image to an electronic version
    b. return all convoluted pixel values back to their original values
    c. change the blacks on an image to white and vice versa
    d. allow image construction in a previous scanning plane

14. **In _____ CT scanning, the table moves continuously through the gantry.**

    a. conventional
    b. spiral
    c. step and shoot
    d. first-generation

15. **Fifth-generation CT scanning is dedicated to imaging (the):**

    a. head
    b. abdominal structures
    c. cardiac system
    d. spine

16. **One major advantage of CT scanning is its:**

    a. high count rate
    b. small pixel sizes
    c. table motion
    d. high contrast resolution

17. **The breakthrough in sixth-generation CT technology that allows for the continuous motion of the patient through the gantry is the use of:**

    a. adjustable collimators
    b. convolution
    c. slip rings
    d. suppression

18. **The scanogram taken during a CT procedure is used to:**

    a. annotate any special windowing used to obtain the images
    b. serve as a scout and reference guide to the section intervals taken
    c. ensure the patient is not wearing any metal objects or other artifact-causing materials
    d. check the linearity of the CT numbers of bone in the image to water

19. **Which of the following will provide the greatest image spatial resolution?**

    a. small pixels, small focal spot size, and narrow collimation
    b. large pixels, higher atomic numbers, and wide collimation
    c. small indexes, faster tube speeds, and large voxels
    d. small voxels, large fields of view, and limited deconvolution

20. To correct for the "cork-screw" image that results due to helical scanning, which of the following image processing tools is used?

    a. reformatting
    b. reverse image
    c. filtering and windowing
    d. interpolation

21. The component of a scintillation detector which is responsible for causing the amplification of the electrons prior to being processed by the computer is the:

    a. photomultiplier tube
    b. dynode
    c. sodium iodide crystal
    d. tungsten plate

22. The collimator determines and/or controls which of the following in CT scanning?

    1. Slice thickness
    2. Patient dose
    3. Table index

    a. 1, 2
    b. 1, 3
    c. 2, 3
    d. 1, 2, 3

23. The CT calibration test which is conducted to ensure that water is consistently represented as zero Hounsfield units is called:

    a. indexing
    b. deconvolution
    c. linearity
    d. line pair measure

24. Image reconstruction in CT scanning relies on which principles?

    1. Filtered back projection
    2. Fourier transform
    3. Iterative reconstruction

    a. 1, 2
    b. 1, 3
    c. 2, 3
    d. 1, 2, 3

25. A broad dark band is apparent on an abdominal CT image. This probably resulted due to:

    a. the presence of metal objects in the scanning field
    b. patient motion
    c. increased beam attenuation through the patient
    d. a detector that has fallen out of calibration

26. Which of the following is the most likely to cause a star artifact?

    a. beam hardening
    b. algorithm errors
    c. tissue averaging
    d. patient jewelry

27. Spatial resolution quality control is conducted:

    a. semiannually by imaging a wire to obtain ERF
    b. daily by imaging a water phantom
    c. annually by imaging a specially designed phantom
    d. semiannually by imaging a resolution test pattern

28. Modern CT scanners have x-ray beams which are:

    a. pencil beams
    b. fan shaped
    c. divergent
    d. helical

29. Each pixel in a CT image is displayed as:

    a. a distinct brightness level
    b. a relative attenuation value
    c. two line pairs
    d. a dotted line on a scanogram

30. If the table movement is equal to the section thickness, then the pitch is:

    a. 100:1
    b. 10:1
    c. 2:1
    d. 1:1

Labeling

1. Identify the components of the CT scanner and the anatomy of the abdominal CT scan.

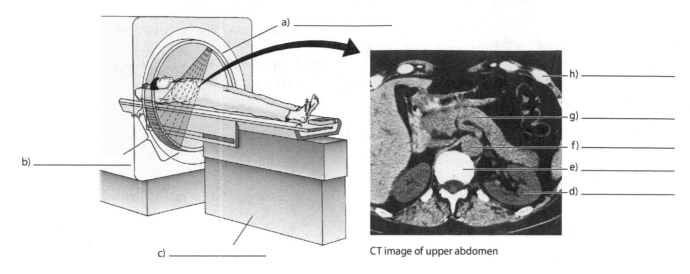

CT image of upper abdomen

a) _____

b) _____

c) _____

h) _____

g) _____

f) _____

e) _____

d) _____

2. Label the lettered components of the scintillation detector.

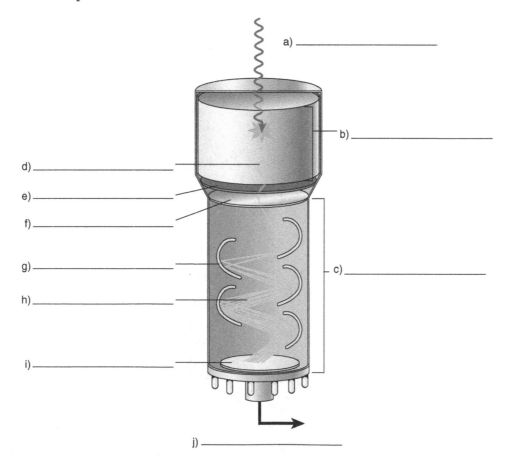

a) _____

b) _____

c) _____

d) _____

e) _____

f) _____

g) _____

h) _____

i) _____

j) _____

3. Complete the table by placing the Hounsfield Unit or CT Number for each tissue type in the appropriate box.

Tissue	Hounsfield Unit or CT Number
Air	_____
Lung	_____
Fat	_____
Water	_____
Tumors	_____
Blood	_____
Cerebrospinal fluid	_____
Gray matter	_____
White matter	_____
Muscle	_____
Liver	_____
Blood, clotted	_____
Dense bone	_____

Crossword Puzzle

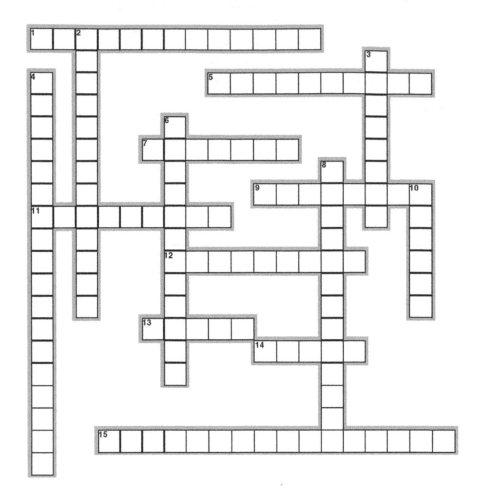

Across

1. This type of detector emits light when struck by x-ray photons
5. This unit assigns specific values to different types of tissue based on their attenuation properties
7. Sixth-generation CT scanners; allows continuous rotation of the x-ray tube and detectors around the patient
9. The positioning of the patient couch; must be reproducible to within 1 mm
11. Term for the scout image of the area to be scanned
12. The mathematical formula performed by the computer that produces the image
13. This ratio is 1:1 if the couch movement is equal to the slice thickness
14. The volume of each pixel element
15. Preferred CT scintillation detector crystal due to its minimal afterglow (two words)

Down

2. Mathematical calculations used to fill in missing data when helical scanning is used
3. These types of objects in the body are responsible for creating star artifacts
4. The ability of a system to distinguish between two objects with similar attenuation values (two words)
6. Using data from a series of images to produce an image in a new scan plane without rescanning the patient
8. Artifact that appears as broad dark bands caused by significant attenuation as it passes through the patient (two words)
10. The doughnut-shaped structure and patient aperture in a CT scanner

PART VI

Radiation Biology and Protection

31

Radiation Biology: Cellular Effects

1. The majority of the human body is made up of:

   a. proteins
   b. water
   c. lipids
   d. carbohydrates

2. The most radiosensitive part of the cell cycle is the ___ phase.

   a. S
   b. G1
   c. M
   d. G2

3. The most radioresistant tissue from the list below is:

   a. lymph
   b. nerve
   c. skin
   d. thyroid

4. The Law of Bergonie and Tribondeau states that:

   1. Younger cells are more radiosensitive
   2. Rapidly dividing cells are more radiosensitive
   3. Mature cells are less radiosensitive
   4. Rapidly growing cells are more radiosensitive

   a. 1, 2
   b. 1, 2, 4
   c. 1, 3, 4
   d. 1, 2, 3, 4

5. The least radioresistant cells in the human body are:

   a. epithelial cells
   b. nerve cells
   c. osteocytes
   d. lymphocytes

6. The technical term for cell division of genetic cells is:

   a. mitosis
   b. meiosis
   c. growth
   d. stochastic

7. Which pairing is not allowed in a DNA molecule?

   a. thymine-cytosine
   b. cystosine-guanine
   c. adenine-thymine
   d. guanine-cytosine

8. The roles of RNA in protein synthesis are:

   a. anabolism and catabolism
   b. osmosis and diffusion
   c. splitting and repairing
   d. copying and translating

189

9. The correct order of mitosis is:

   a. telophase, anaphase, metaphase, and prophase
   b. anaphase, metaphase, prophase, and inter-
      phase
   c. prophase, metaphase, anaphase, and telophase
   d. interphase, telophase, prophase, and meta-
      phase

10. An indirect effect of radiation exposure to the
    cell involves the:

    a. DNA bond
    b. cell membrane
    c. cytoplasm
    d. organelles

11. The number of chromosomes that result in each
    daughter cell after meiosis is:

    a. 2
    b. 12
    c. 23
    d. 46

12. DNA duplication occurs during which phase of
    the cell cycle?

    a. prophase
    b. metaphase
    c. S phase
    d. G1

13. The cell component that digests macromole-
    cules to produce energy is the:

    a. ribosomes
    b. endoplasmic reticulum
    c. lysosomes
    d. mitochondria

14. Each amino acid is manufactured from three
    base pairs in a series called (a/n):

    a. codon
    b. triton
    c. organelle
    d. mutation

15. Ionizing radiation is able to produce which one
    of the following effects?

    1. Cell death
    2. Cancer
    3. Free radicals

    a. 1, 2
    b. 1, 3
    c. 2, 3
    d. 1, 2, 3

16. Chromatin condenses into visible chromosomes
    during which phase of mitosis?

    a. interphase
    b. prophase
    c. metaphase
    d. telophase

17. Which of the following types of radiation has the
    highest LET?

    a. gamma rays
    b. bremsstrahlung
    c. alpha particles
    d. x-rays

18. Immature somatic cells are called:

    a. germ cells
    b. stem cells
    c. genetic cells
    d. oogonia

19. The factor that would increase a cell's radiosen-
    sitivity and chance of cell death is:

    a. fractionation of the dose
    b. the presence of oxygen
    c. lower RBE radiation
    d. H− and OH+ combining to H_2O

20. The formula, D_{250}/D_r, is used to calculate:

    a. RBE
    b. LET
    c. R_W
    d. OER

21. Based on the Law of Bergonie and Tribondeau, which type of cells would be more radiosensitive?

    a. neurons
    b. chondrocytes
    c. erythroblasts
    d. myocytes

22. Lipids would be the most likely to be found in which part of the cell?

    a. membrane
    b. nucleolus
    c. ribosomes
    d. centromere

23. The target theory states that if ionization occurs in or near a key molecule:

    a. enzymes and proteins will be irreparably damaged
    b. restitutions is still highly likely
    c. DNA may be inactivated and the cell will die
    d. two ion pairs and two free radicals are produced

24. All of the following are factors that can affect radiosensitivity except:

    a. RBE
    b. OER
    c. LET
    d. OH

25. How does the linear energy transfer (LET) of a radiation affect its relative biologic effectiveness (RBE)?

    a higher LET radiations have higher RBE values
    b. higher LET radiations have lower RBE values
    c. higher LET radiations cause RBE to stabilize
    d. lower LET radiations cause RBE to stabilize

26. The indirect effect is the most likely to result in which of the following?

    a. amino acids
    b. H_2O_2 and free radicals
    c. broken DNA bonds
    d. excess oxygen

27. Which of the following are functions of proteins in the body?

    1. Antibodies
    2. Enzymes
    3. Hormones

    a. 1, 2
    b. 1, 3
    c. 2, 3
    d. 1, 2, 3

28. Glucose would be classified as a:

    a. monosaccharide
    b. lipid
    c. organelle
    d. amino acid

29. The differences between RNA and DNA are:

    1. DNA has two strands and RNA has one
    2. DNA plays a role in gene function and protein function
    3. DNA is found only in the cytoplasm and RNA in the nucleolus

    a. 1, 2
    b. 1, 3
    c. 2, 3
    d. 1, 2, 3

30. Based upon the Law of Bergonie and Tribondeau, the fetus is highly radiosensitive because of:

    a. low rate of proliferation
    b. high rate of mitotic activity
    c. large numbers of mature and highly differentiated cells
    d. its environment

Labeling

1. Label the lettered cell components.

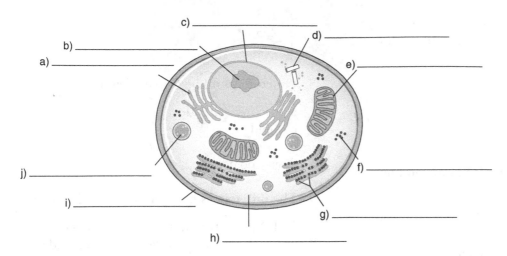

2. Identify each phase in the cell division process of mitosis.

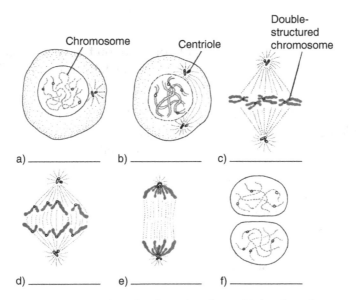

Modified from Sadler T. W. *Langman's Medical Embryology.* 12th ed. Baltimore, MD: Lippincott Williams & Wilkins, 2012, with permission.

3. Label the various results due to the radiolysis of water.

H_2O

a)_____
_____

HOH^+
HOH^-

b)_____
_____

H^+
H^-

c)_____
_____

OH^*
H^*

$OH^* + OH^* = H_2O_2$

d)_____
_____

4. Complete the table by listing the cells and organs which are assigned to each category of radiosensitivity: most, intermediate, and least.

Most sensitive   _____
                      _____
                      _____
                      _____
                      _____

Intermediate   _____
                      _____
                      _____
                      _____
                      _____
                      _____

Least sensitive   _____
                      _____
                      _____
                      _____

Crossword Puzzle

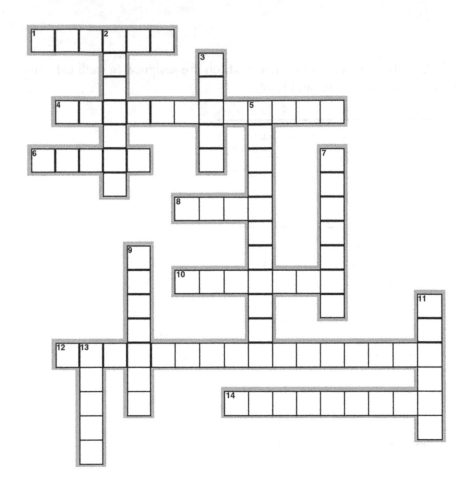

Across

1. This theory suggests that for a cell to die after irradiation, a key molecule must be inactivated
4. Results after the indirect effect has occurred in addition to hydrogen peroxide (two words)
6. Eighty percent of the human body is made of this substance
8. Newly formed, immature cells; _____ cells
10. The reduction and division process for genetic cells
12. Term used to describe a cell's or organ's ability to be damaged by radiation
14. The stage of mitosis where the chromosomes are aligned across the spindle of the nucleus

Down

2. Type of cells produced by the reproductive organs
3. Term for a series of three base pairs; used in the manufacture of amino acids and proteins
5. Each normal human somatic cell has 46 of these
7. A monosaccharide
9. The purine that pairs with thymine in a DNA molecule
11. Radiosensitivity is increased when this gaseous element is present
13. A high LET radiation

Organism Response to Radiation

32

1. The dose-response relationship upon which all of our radiation protection procedures are based upon is:

   a. nonlinear threshold
   b. linear threshold
   c. linear nonthreshold
   d. sigmoid threshold

2. A deterministic (or nonstochastic) effect is associated the most closely with:

   a. early effects of human responses to radiation exposure
   b. late effects of human responses to radiation exposure
   c. low doses of radiation fractionated over time
   d. low doses of radiation received later in life

3. Which of the following physical effects follows a threshold nonlinear response?

   a. life span shortening
   b. cancer
   c. epilation
   d. genetic mutations

4. Fever, faintness, and nausea are symptoms principally associated with which stage of ARS?

   a. recovery
   b. latent period
   c. prodromal
   d. manifest illness

5. Between 10 and 50 Gy (1,000 to 5,000 rads) of acute radiation exposure, the systems affected during the manifest illness period are the:

   1. Hematopoietic system
   2. GI system
   3. CNS system

   a. 3 only
   b. 1, 2
   c. 2, 3
   d. 1, 2, 3

6. A radiation victim presents with the following symptoms: Nausea, confusion, headache, slurred speech, and delirium. The dose this patient was probably exposed to was:

   a. less than 1 Gy (100 rad)
   b. 2 to 10 Gy (200 to 1,000 rad)
   c. 10 to 50 Gy (1,000 to 5,000 rad)
   d. 50 Gy or more (5,000+ rad)

7. The stage of high-dose radiation effects in which the individual appears to have recovered but may still exhibit symptoms at a later date is called the:

   a. prodromal stage
   b. latent period
   c. acute stage
   d. recovery stage

8. The high-dose effect occurring at doses from 1 to 6 Gy (100 to 600 rads) is the:

   a. prodromal stage
   b. hematologic syndrome
   c. gastrointestinal syndrome
   d. central nervous syndrome

9. In general, the length (course) of acute radiation syndrome:

   a. decreases with increasing dose
   b. is affected only by the type of radiation exposure received
   c. relatively constant and predictable at all dose levels
   d. increases with increasing dose

10. When evaluating a cell survival curve, a curve with a wider shoulder portion would indicate:

    a. at least 37% of the cells have died
    b. an increased lethality
    c. a higher ratio of survival
    d. a higher LET radiation was used

11. The D_Q in the cell survival curve describes the:

    a. number of targets actually hit
    b. organelle damage
    c. DNA damage
    d. threshold dose of the irradiated cells

12. If an effect is considered to be a threshold effect, this means that:

    a. any dose of radiation is unsafe
    b. once humans reach a certain age, their radiosensitivity decreases
    c. a minimum dose must be reached before the effect is seen
    d. it is either there or not (an "all or none" response)

13. The linear nonthreshold dose-response model is more closely associated with:

    a. stochastic effects
    b. somatic effects
    c. deterministic effects
    d. ARS effects

14. Higher doses result in _____ latent periods.

    a. shorter
    b. longer
    c. unchanged
    d. none of the above

15. Ionizing radiation is a/n:

    a. carcinogen
    b. lysosome
    c. pyrimidine
    d. annihilator

16. The doubling dose for genetic effects is from _____.

    a. 0.01 to 0.1 Gy (1 and 10 rads)
    b. 0.5 to 1.0 Gy (50 and 100 rads)
    c. 2.0 to 4.0 Gy (200 and 400 rads)
    d. 5 to 10 Gy (500 and 1,000 rads)

17. The skin erythema dose (SED 50) is approximately:

    a. 0.5 Gy (50 rads)
    b. 1 Gy (100 rads)
    c. 3 Gy (300 rads)
    d. 6 Gy (600 rads)

18. The dose to produce epilation to the scalp is approximately:

    a. 0.5 Gy (50 rads)
    b. 1 Gy (100 rads)
    c. 3 Gy (300 rads)
    d. 6 Gy (600 rads)

19. The $LD_{50/30}$ dose to the whole body with no medical support is approximately:

    a. 0.5 Gy (50 rads)
    b. 1 Gy (100 rads)
    c. 3 Gy (300 rads)
    d. 6 Gy (600 rads)

20. The term epilation is used to refer to:

    a. loss of hair
    b. lower white blood cell formation
    c. metabolism
    d. cataract formation

21. Teratogenic effects result when:

    a. an oocyte is irradiated prior to conception
    b. a fetus is exposed to radiation in utero
    c. the gonadal dose reaches 2 Gy
    d. all three ARS syndrome are present concurrently

22. If a fetus is irradiated at approximately 7 weeks' gestation, the most likely effect would be:

    a. leukemia in early childhood
    b. spontaneous abortion
    c. anophthalmia
    d. no effect

23. Once the fetus reaches the 16th week of gestation:

    a. radiosensitivity matches that of an adult
    b. mental retardation is a likely effect if irradiation occurs at this stage
    c. spontaneous abortion risk increases with in utero exposures
    d. latent carcinogenic effects are more likely with fetal exposure

24. Genetic effects of radiation are associated with:

    a. RBE
    b. OER
    c. LET
    d. GSD

25. Mutagenic or genetic effects are more likely to occur if:

    a. the fetus is irradiated
    b. skin dose reaches desquamation levels
    c. the gonads are exposed to the primary beam
    d. the radiation dose is protracted

26. Cancer and genetic effects are examples of _____ effects.

    a. stochastic
    b. nonstochastic
    c. threshold
    d. acute radiation syndrome

27. Which of the following populations have experienced an excess incidence of bone cancers?

    a. uranium miners
    b. radium watch dial painters
    c. Chernobyl victims
    d. radiologic technologists

28. The stages of acute radiation syndrome in order are:

    a. prodromal, latent, manifest, recovery/death
    b. prodromal, manifest, latent, recovery/death
    c. manifest, latent, prodromal, recovery/death
    d. latent, manifest, prodromal, recovery/death

29. Which of the following physiological effects are associated with and the most likely to occur as a result of a patient who is a victim of the hematopoietic syndrome of acute radiation syndrome?

    a. decreased leukocytes and thrombocytes
    b. nausea and bloody diarrhea
    c. thrombus formation and remission
    d. headaches and coma

30. Based upon the Law of Bergonie and Tribondeau, the fetus is highly radiosensitive because of:

    a. low rate of proliferation
    b. high rate of mitotic activity
    c. large numbers of mature and highly differentiated cells
    d. its environment

Labeling

1. Identify and label each component of the cell survival curve.

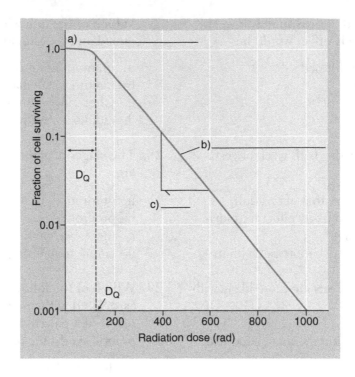

2. Evaluate each dose-response curve and determine whether it is linear or nonlinear and threshold or nonthreshold.

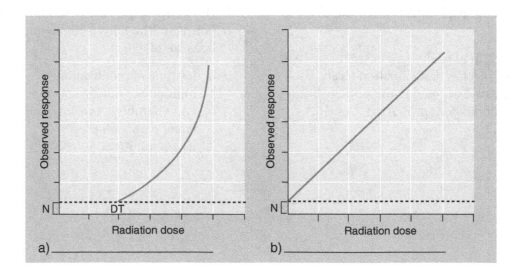

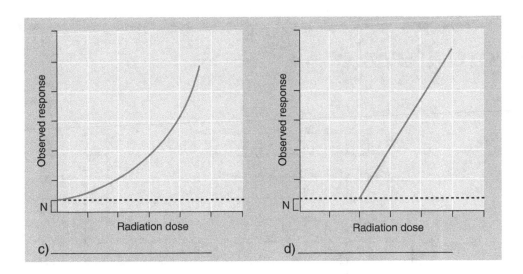

3. Identify the dose rate, latency period, and average time period for each syndrome associated with Acute Radiation Syndrome.

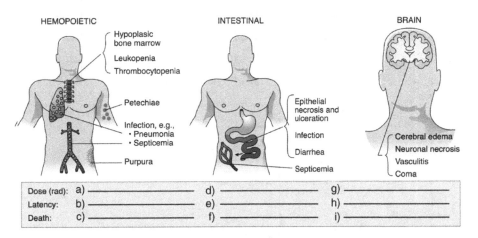

(Modified from Rubin E, Strayer, DS. Rubin's Pathology: Clinicopathologic Foundations of Medicine. 7th ed. Philadelphia, PA: Wolters Kluwer Health, 2015.)

Crossword Puzzle

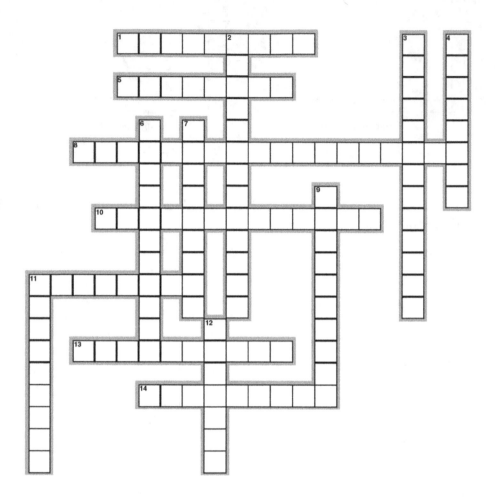

Across

1. The minimum dose needed for a specific effect to become evident
5. Cancer of the blood due to bone marrow irradiation
8. The dose-response curve that BEIR has used to determine current radiation protection guidelines
10. An effect or response not observed until a minimum dose is reached; the magnitude of the effect increases with increasing dose
11. Skin reddening due to radiation exposure
13. The term applied to any factor or activity that can cause cancer
14. A radiation effect on the chromosomes of human gametes prior to fertilization

Down

2. The ARS syndrome that occurs between 1 and 6 Gy whole body exposure; causes a decrease in erythrocytes and leukocytes
3. The stage of gestation between 2 and 8 weeks where radiation exposure could lead to skeletal or neurologic defects in the fetus
4. Region of the cell survival curve that indicates the amount of cell repair or recovery
6. The classification of effects that occur due to irradiation of a fetus in utero
7. The first stage of acute radiation syndrome
9. The type of radiation effect that occurs randomly and has an "all or none" response
11. Hair loss due to radiation exposure
12. Cataracts are an example of a late _____ effect

33

Radiation Protection: Principle Concepts and Equipment

1. The major component of radiation exposure due to man-made sources is:

   a. nuclear power plants
   b. natural gas
   c. nuclear weapons fallout
   d. medical sources

2. The major component of radiation exposure due to natural sources is:

   a. cosmic
   b. radon
   c. internal (C-14)
   d. consumer products

3. Three sources of natural background radiation are:

   a. cosmic, polyurethanes, and internal
   b. atmospheric, extraneous, and electrical
   c. internal, terrestrial, and cosmic
   d. medical, consumer products, and radon

4. In general, radiation doses to the U.S. population:

   a. have decreased due to the greater use of nonionizing diagnostic exams such as MRI and ultrasound
   b. have increased due to the increased use of computed tomography in the last 30 years
   c. have decreased due to better equipment and the use of digital imaging methods
   d. have increased due to the increased use of nuclear power worldwide

5. What is the unit of absorbed dose in the SI system?

   a. Curie
   b. rad
   c. rem
   d. Gray

6. Effective dose is calculated to determine:

   a. the amount of radioactivity present in an isotope
   b. the number of ionizations present in air
   c. the relative risk of the dose received by various tissues
   d. the energy of an x-ray photon

7. The annual effective dose limit for an occupationally exposed radiation worker is:

   a. 5 mSv (0.5 rems)
   b. 50 mSv (5 rems)
   c. 1 mSv (0.1 rem)
   d. 10 mSv (1 rem)

8. The cumulative effective dose limit for a 25-year-old radiographer is:

   a. 25 mSv
   b. 50 mSV
   c. 100 mSv
   d. 250 mSv

9. A personnel monitor report would express a radiographer's dose equivalent in:

   a. Becquerels (Curies)
   b. C/kg (Roentgens)
   c. mSv (mrem)
   d. mGy (mrad)

10. The tissue with the highest tissue weighting factor (as developed by the ICRP) of those listed below is:

    a. breast
    b. thyroid
    c. bone marrow
    d. gonads

11. The principle that states that patient and personnel exposure should reduced as much as possible is often referred to as:

    a. LET
    b. RBE
    c. NCRP
    d. ALARA

12. Occupationally exposed workers must wear a personnel monitor if _____ of the annual dose equivalent limit could be received.

    a. 1/10
    b. ¼
    c. ½
    d. 100%

13. The longest interval that a personnel monitor should be worn is:

    a. 1 week
    b. 1 month
    c. 3 months
    d. 1 year

14. Which of the following statements best describes effective dose?

    a. the lethal dose to humans if received in one whole-body exposure
    b. the dose received by the patient at the skin level
    c. the dose that accounts for biologic harm as a result of the body part that is exposed and the type of radiation used
    d. the dose of any exam as compared to a chest x-ray

15. To calculate the effective dose received by a specific organ, the absorbed dose value is:

    a. added to the tissue weighting factor
    b. multiplied by the tissue weighting factor
    c. subtracted from the tissue weighting factor
    d. divided by the tissue weighting factor

16. Which of the following radiations has the lowest radiation weighting factor?

    a. x-rays
    b. neutrons
    c. protons
    d. alpha

17. The detector that requires heating to obtain a dose reading is the:

    a. gas-filled detector
    b. scintillator
    c. TLD
    d. GM counter

18. The detector that is used to calibrate and evaluate x-ray unit performance is the:

    a. gas-filled detector
    b. scintillator
    c. TLD
    d. GM counter

19. The type of radiation detector that gives off light when struck by radiation are called:

    a. gas-filled
    b. GM counters
    c. scintillation detectors
    d. prereading dosimeters

20. Radiation workers must wear a personnel monitor device:

    1. daily
    2. at the hip level
    3. on the anterior surface of the body

    a. 1, 2
    b. 1, 3
    c. 2, 3
    d. 1, 2, 3

21. The most commonly used crystal used in a thermoluminescent dosimeter that "stores" the exposure for later reading is:

    a. calcium tungstate
    b. lithium fluoride
    c. cesium iodide
    d. aluminum oxide

22. The most sensitive type of personnel monitoring devices available because of their ability to detect exposures as low as 1 mrem are:

    a. film badges
    b. GM counters
    c. optically stimulated luminescent devices
    d. monthly blood tests

23. The smallest practical dose that a standard film badge can measure is approximately:

    a. 1.0 mrem (0.01 mSv)
    b. 10 mrem (0.1 mSv)
    c. 25 mrem (0.25 mSv)
    d. 100 mrem (1 mSv)

24. Which of the following is NOT a basic component of a film badge?

    a. silver halide emulsion
    b. copper filters
    c. cadmium filters
    d. self-reading meter

25. The personnel monitoring device that allows the worker to read his/her dose at the end of each workday is the:

    a. film badge
    b. TLD
    c. OSL
    d. Instadose

26. The general public's effective dose limit is approximately _____ of the occupationally exposed workers.

    a. 1/100
    b. 1/10
    c. ¼
    d. ½

27. A scintillation detector would be used in which of the following medical imaging applications?

    1. MRI
    2. CT
    3. Nuclear Medicine

    a. 1, 2
    b. 1, 3
    c. 2, 3
    d. 1, 2, 3

28. The allowable annual dose limit to a radiation worker's hands is:

    a. 50 mSv
    b. 150 mSv
    c. 300 mSv
    d. 500 mSv

29. The organization which recommends dose limits (DLs) in the United States for radiation workers is the:

    a. NCRP
    b. NRC
    c. ARRT
    d. ICRP

30. When whole-body occupational exposure is controlled by keeping the effective absorbed dose equivalent well below the upper boundary limit, the possibility of causing stochastic effects of radiation is:

    a. increased
    b. only double that of the general population
    c. minimized
    d. totally eliminated

Labeling

1. Complete the table of radiation units by placing the SI and conventional units and their ratios in their appropriate boxes.

Quantity	SI Unit	Conventional Unit	Ratio of SI to Conventional
Exposure	_____	_____	_____
Dose	_____	_____	_____
Effective dose	_____	_____	_____
Activity	_____	_____	_____

2. Complete the table listing the radiation weighting factor assigned to each type of radiation.

Type and Energy Range	Radiation Weighting Factor (W_r)
X- and gamma rays, electrons	_____
Neutrons, energy <10 keV	_____
10–100 keV	_____
>100 keV–2 MeV	_____
>2–20 MeV	_____
>20 MeV	_____
Protons	_____
Alpha particles	_____

3. Complete the table identifying the dose limit set for each radiation worker factor listed.

	Dose Limit Values
Occupational Exposures	
Effective dose limits	
a. Annual	_____
b. Cumulative	_____
Equivalent annual dose limits for tissues and organs	
a. Lens of the eye	_____
b. Skin, hands, and feet, red bone marrow and thyroid	_____
Education and Training Exposures (Annual)	
Effective dose limit	_____
Equivalent dose limits for tissues and organs	
a. Lens of the eye	_____
b. Skin, hands, and feet	_____
Embryo/Fetus Exposures	
a. Total equivalent dose limit	_____
b. Monthly equivalent dose limit	_____
Negligible Individual Dose (annual)	_____
Public Exposure (annual)	
Effective dose limit	
a. Exposure	_____
Equivalent dose limits for tissues and organs	
a. Lens of the eye	_____
b. Skin, hands, and feet	_____

Crossword Puzzle

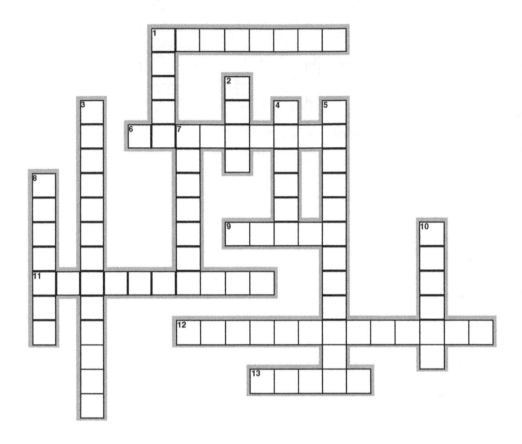

Across

1. Conventional unit of exposure
6. Type of personnel monitor that is an active ion and USB device; allows immediate reporting of dose using a computer
9. Type of light used to stimulate the emission of an OSL crystal
11. The dose limit calculated using the formula: age × 10 mSv
12. Type of radiation detector that emits light when struck by radiation; _____ detector
13. As low as reasonably achievable

Down

1. A terrestrial source of exposure; a radioactive gas
2. SI unit for absorbed dose
3. Radiosensitive crystal used in an OSL personnel monitor (two words)
4. The most radiosensitive tissue based on its tissue weighting factor (Wt) of 0.20
5. Gas-filled survey meter (hyphen.)
7. SI unit of effective dose
8. The primary source of man-made radiation exposure in the United States
10. Source of natural radiation exposure from outer space

34

Minimizing Exposure to Ionizing Radiation

1. The radiation exposure to the technologist and radiologist can be decreased by reducing the:

   a. fluoroscopy time
   b. distance
   c. shielding
   d. monitor badge

2. Increasing the distance from the patient will:

   a. increase the scattered radiation reaching the staff
   b. decrease the time of radiation exposure
   c. decrease the scattered radiation reaching the staff
   d. none of the above

3. Which of the following is the source of scattered radiation during a fluoroscopy procedure?

   a. the operator
   b. the patient
   c. the image intensifier
   d. the table

4. What percent of scatter radiation do lead aprons attenuate?

   a. 10%
   b. 50%
   c. 80%
   d. 99%

5. Which of the following technical factors can reduce radiation dose to the patient?

   a. low mAs, long time
   b. high kVp, low mAs
   c. low kVp, high mAs
   d. high kVp, high mAs

6. Lead aprons, when not in use, should be placed:

   a. in a heap
   b. on hanging racks
   c. folded twice and put away
   d. stuffed in a container

7. Lead aprons and other protective apparel should be inspected for cracks by:

   1. Visual inspection
   2. Using a radiation dosimeter
   3. Using fluoroscopy

   a. 1, 2
   b. 1, 3
   c. 2, 3
   d. 1, 2, 3

8. The technologist is allowed to hold a patient during an exposure:

   a. when the patient is in danger of falling
   b. when the patient is a baby
   c. when the patient is in pain
   d. never

9. According to the inverse square law, if a technologist doubles the distance she is standing from the radiation source, her dose will:

   a. decrease to ½
   b. decrease to ¼
   c. increase two times
   d. increase four times

10. The type of gonadal shielding that is suspended from the collimator:

    a. flat contact
    b. lead apron
    c. shadow
    d. lead strip

11. The monthly effective dose limit for a declared pregnant technologist is:

    a. 0.5 mSv
    b. 5.0 mSv
    c. 50 mSv
    d. 500 mSv

12. If the x-ray tube's peak energy can reach 100 kVp, lead aprons must have a minimum thickness of:

    a. 2.5 mm Al
    b. 0.25 mm Pb
    c. 0.5 mm Al
    d. 0.5 mm Pb

13. Compared to the primary beam, scatter radiation is _____.

    a. 100 times more intense
    b. 100 times less intense
    c. 1,000 times more intense
    d. 1,000 times less intense

14. Who would be the best individual to help hold a patient who is unsteady on her feet during an x-ray exposure?

    a. the patient's husband
    b. the technologist
    c. the radiologist
    d. the patient's pregnant daughter

15. If the technique used for an x-ray exposure is changed from 20 mAs to 40 mAs, the patient dose will:

    a. increase 2 times
    b. decrease 2 times
    c. remain unchanged
    d. change only if kVp is changed, also

16. Which of the following radiographic examinations would cause the highest entrance skin exposure (ESE)?

    a. pediatric chest x-ray
    b. PA adult chest x-ray
    c. a finger exam
    d. a lumbar spine exam

17. Which of the following actions would limit the radiation exposure to the radiologist and the technologist during fluoroscopy?

    1. Use of intermittent fluoro
    2. Pulsed fluoroscopy
    3. Continuous exposure fluoro

    a. 1, 2
    b. 1, 3
    c. 2, 3
    d. 1, 2, 3

18. The second fetal personnel monitor issued to a declared pregnant worker should be worn:

    a. at the collar level
    b. as a ring badge
    c. at waist level
    d. directly over the fetus

19. The purpose of "The Ten Day Rule" is to:

    a. prohibit all x-ray examinations on women of childbearing age until 10 days after menses to protect an unsuspected fetus
    b. ensure that childbearing women do not have any abdominal or pelvic examinations during the menstrual period
    c. limit abdominal and pelvic region examinations to the first 10 days of the menstrual cycle to protect an unsuspected fetus
    d. allow women of childbearing age up to 10 days to schedule all abdomen/pelvic x-ray examination

20. During a fluoroscopic examination, which of the following would be the BEST place for the radiographer to stand in order to minimize his/her exposure?

    a. as close as possible to the examining table
    b. as far away as practical from the examining table
    c. at the patient's head
    d. facing away from the fluoro tower and image intensifier

21. The TVL value is used to determine:

    a. occupational dose
    b. adequate filtration
    c. occupancy factor
    d. primary and secondary barriers

22. Which of the following is/are classified as (a) controlled area(s)?

    a. radiographic room
    b. hallway
    c. unattended elevators
    d. waiting room

23. Secondary barriers serve to shield for _____ radiation.

    1. Leakage
    2. Scatter
    3. Direct

    a. 1, 2
    b. 1, 3
    c. 2, 3
    d. 1, 2, 3

24. When planning protection for a diagnostic x-ray installation, the workload (w) is usually stated in:

    a. Roentgens-mA/week
    b. mA-min/week
    c. heat units (HU)/week
    d. kV-mA min/week

25. Protective lead barriers must extend _____ up from the floor.

    a. 5 feet
    b. 7 feet
    c. 10 feet
    d. always to ceiling height

26. The wall upon which the vertical bucky is mounted must contain:

    a. 2.5 mm Al equivalent
    b. 1/32" (0.79 mm) Pb equivalent
    c. 1/16" (1.58 mm) Pb equivalent
    d. 0.5 mm Pb equivalent

27. A cumulative timing device runs during the x-ray exposure and sounds an audible alarm or temporarily interrupts the exposure after the fluoroscope has been activated for:

    a. 30 seconds
    b. 2 minutes
    c. 5 minutes
    d. 10 minutes

28. Which of the following actions will reduce repeat exposures?

    a. increasing the SID
    b. light field/x-ray field alignment
    c. asking for the possibility of pregnancy prior to an examination
    d. increasing the exposure time during pediatric examinations

29. The control booth is considered both a controlled area and:

    a. must be designed as a secondary barrier
    b. is placed on the same wall as the chest bucky
    c. is designed so that the technologist can peer around the corner to ensure the patient's safety
    d. must therefore automatically contain 1.58 mm Pb

30. Which of the following technologist practices do not meet ALARA guidelines?

    a. providing clear instructions and using short exposure times
    b. wearing a lead apron during portable examinations
    c. consistently using increased mAs values with CR/DR systems
    d. immobilizing a pediatric patient during a routine chest exam

Labeling

1. For each lettered item, label the type of radiation being emitted and identify whether it is considered primary or secondary radiation.

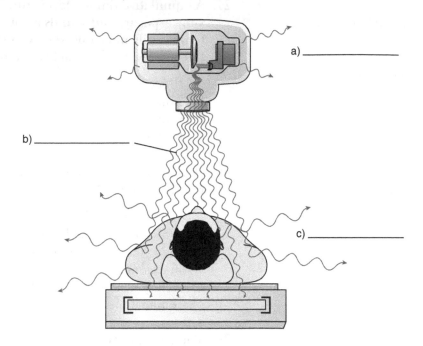

a) _____

b) _____

c) _____

2. Evaluate the radiographic room layout and determine whether Wall A and Wall B are primary or a secondary barriers. Also list the amount of lead that should be present in each barrier. Write your answers in the blank spaces provided.

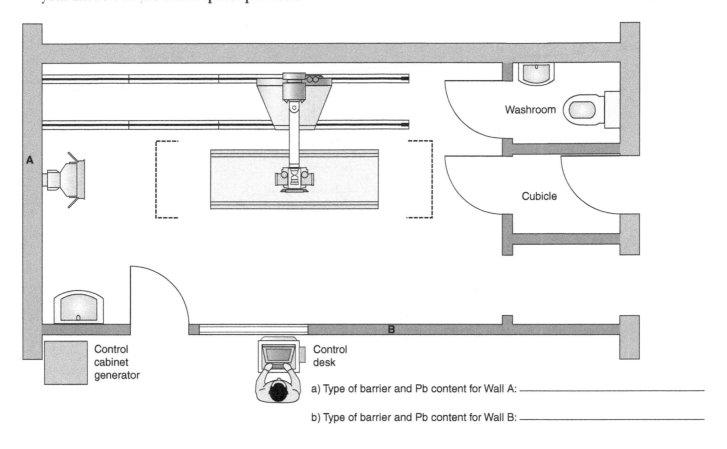

a) Type of barrier and Pb content for Wall A: _____

b) Type of barrier and Pb content for Wall B: _____

3. Identify the different exposure levels to the radiographer when distance is changed

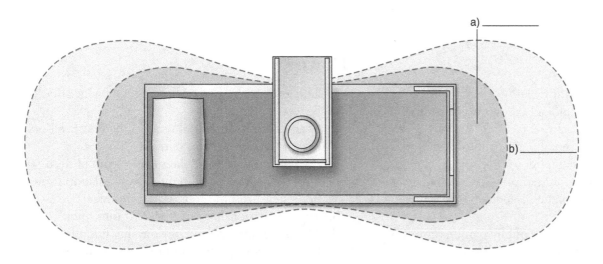

Crossword Puzzle

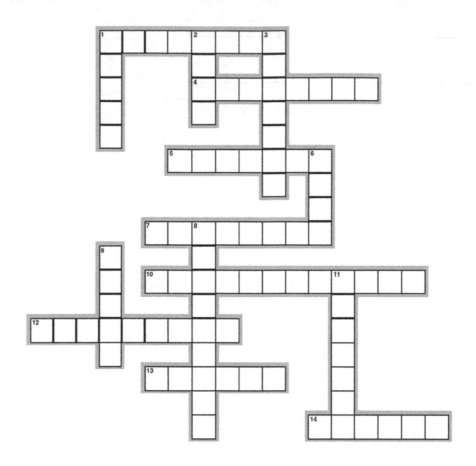

Across

1. Measured in mA-min/wk
4. The frequency that lead aprons are inspected for cracks
5. The primary source of scatter and occupational dose for the radiographer
7. One of the three cardinal principles of radiation protection; best practice is to keep this as great as possible
10. Areas where the general public can be found; includes waiting rooms and hallways
12. One of the three cardinal principles of radiation protection; involves using a barrier
13. Type of gonadal shield that is suspended from the collimator
14. The rule that states all elective abdominal radiographs on women of childbearing age should be postponed until this period (two words)

Down

1. The level of the body where a fetal badge should be worn
2. Most common material used in the construction of radiation protection barriers
3. Each repeat exposure does this to patient dose
6. One of the three cardinal rules of radiation protection; measured in seconds and minutes
8. Type of barrier that must be 0.79 mm thick
9. The designated period of time that it is allowable for a technologist to stand in the primary beam
11. Type of unwanted radiation from the tube housing

Laboratory
Experiments

Electric and Magnetic Fields

Name: _____ Date: _____

Electrostatics is the study of stationary or resting electric charges. An electric field exists around all electric charges. An English scientist, Michael Faraday (1791 to 1867), introduced the concept of using lines of force as an aid in visualizing the magnitude and direction of an electric field. Similarly, the magnetic force per unit pole is called the magnetic field. In this case, the field is mapped out by using the poles of magnets. The purpose of this activity is to allow the student to visualize and map both electric and magnetic fields and compare their similarities and differences.

Objectives:

Upon completion of this lab, the student will be able to:

1. Draw the electric field surrounding both positive and negative charges
2. Visualize and draw the magnetic field surrounding magnets
3. Apply the laws of electrostatic and magnetic fields to his/her drawing
4. Compare and contrast the similarities and differences in electric and magnetic fields and their respective laws of interaction

Part I: Electrostatic Fields

Draw the electric fields for each charge configuration below, indicating the lines of force, and/or their interactions as applicable. After you have completed your sketches, answer the questions.

A. The Electric Field of a Single Point Charge

$\oplus$

B. The Electric Field of Two Like Point Charges

$\oplus$ $\oplus$

C. The Electric Field of Two Unlike Point Charges

$\oplus$ $\ominus$

1. What are the main differences between Items B and C? What law of electrostatics is illustrated in both of these situations?

_____

_____

_____

2. In situation C, if the force represented at the current distance is equal to 3.0 N, what would be the new force if the distance between the charges was increased? Complete the sentence below with your answer.

   If the distances between the charges is increased, then the force of the _____ (attraction/repulsion) will be _____(increased/decreased).
   a. Whose law is being applied here?

_____

_____

_____

Part II: Magnetic Fields

Materials:

1. Two bar magnets
2. Iron filings
3. Paper

Procedure:

1. Cover the bar magnets with a sheet of paper in the following configurations:
   a. A single bar magnet
   b. Two bar magnets with the North and South poles next to each other with ~ 5 cm separating each magnetic pole
   c. Two bar magnets with the South and South poles next to each other with ~ 5 cm apart separating each magnetic pole

2. Sprinkle an ample amount of iron filings on top of the paper in order to obtain a visible pattern of the magnetic field.

3. Sketch the observed magnetic field patterns for each configuration, rendering the field lines as close to actual size as possible.

4. After the patterns have been sketched, collect the iron filings using your paper as a "funnel" and return them to the container (recycling them for someone else's use).

5. Complete your sketches by indicating the direction of the magnetic field lines. Attach your drawings to this lab report, and answer the following questions.

Analysis:

1. Look at your drawing for the single bar magnet. What happens to the distance between the field lines as the distance increases from the magnet?

_____

_____

_____

2. Evaluate the difference in the magnetic fields for configurations b and c. What law of magnetism is being illustrated?

_____

_____

_____

3. If the magnets in configuration b were moved farther apart, what would happen to the force of attraction/repulsion? Whose law would be illustrated in this case?

_____

_____

_____

4. Compare the electric and magnetic field arrangements you sketched. Describe the differences and similarities between the fields and the laws that they obey?

_____

_____

_____

5. What is one fundamental difference between electric charges versus magnetic poles?

_____

_____

_____

Faraday's Law

Name: _____   **Date:** _____

Michael Faraday is credited with discovering electromagnetic induction: when a wire moves or magnetic field changes so that the flux (field) lines are cut by the wire, an EMF will be induced in the wire. Electromagnetic induction is an important fundamental principle, because it is the basis for the operation of various components in the x-ray tube and circuit.

Faraday's law explains that the induced voltage (EMF) in a coil is proportional to the product of the number of loops and the rate at which the magnetic field changes within the loops. This lab provides students with the opportunity to test various aspects of Faraday's law and observe the effects of electromagnetic induction.

Objectives:

Upon the completion of this lab, the student will be able to:

1. Describe the conditions that must be present in order for electromagnetic induction to occur
2. Demonstrate and describe the following aspects of Faraday's law:
   a) Demonstrate and describe the type of motion necessary to induce voltage using a conductor and a magnet
   b) Determine what effects the number of loops and motion have on the amount of voltage induced

Materials:

1. Galvanometer
2. Bar magnet
3. Long solenoid
4. Short solenoid
5. Black and red connecting wires

Procedure:

1. Connect the positive and negative ends of the galvanometer to the positive and negative ends of the long solenoid. When connected correctly, the galvanometer should register current when the magnet is moved inside the galvanometer. Follow the instructions and answer the questions as indicated.

Data and Analysis:

1. Insert the bar magnet into the coil. What happened to the needle/display? What does the galvanometer register?

_____

_____

_____

2. Leave the magnet stationary inside the coil. What does the galvanometer read now?

_____

_____

_____

3. Slide the magnet back and forth repeatedly inside the coil. Document the galvanometer results.

_____

_____

_____

4. Move the magnet up and down repeatedly inside the coil. Record the galvanometer results.

_____

_____

_____

5. Hold the magnet stationary. Rapidly move the coil back and forth around the magnet. Record the galvanometer readings.

_____

_____

_____

6. Connect the short solenoid coil to the galvanometer using the same connections outlined in the Procedures section. Repeat Step 3. Record the new galvanometer readings. How does this value compare with the longer solenoid?

_____

_____

_____

7. Based on your results above, what conditions must exist in order to produce voltage and current according to Faraday's law? (List all that apply)

_____

_____

_____

Effect of Technical Factors on X-Ray Beam Intensity and Exposure Indicator Numbers

Name: _____   Date: _____

The primary technical factors that a technologist uses to ensure a proper exposure and appearance of the image are mA, time, and kVp. Each of these factors can be changed independently, and each has an effect on the total exposure received by the patient and the image receptor. As a result, each therefore affects the exposure indicator number of the digital imaging system being used. It is essential that a technologist understand the effect that each technique change has on the x-ray beam's quantity and the subsequent effect this has on the exposure indicator number. Understanding this relationship provides the technologist with the ability to apply the proper technique rules if corrective factors are needed in the case of an improperly exposed image.

Objectives:

Upon completion of this lab, the student will be able to:

1. Independently set kVp, time, and mA
2. Properly use an ionization chamber or R-meter to measure x-ray machine output
3. Evaluate the effect of technique changes on radiographic images
4. Evaluate the effect of technique changes on exposure indicator numbers
5. Synthesize the relationships between the technique changes and the visual image changes and the exposure number changes

Materials:

1. Energized radiographic unit
2. R-meter or ionization chamber
3. Computed radiographic unit or DR unit
4. Knee phantom
5. Lead markers to number each exposure

Procedure:

1. Place the knee phantom in an AP position and expose using a bucky technique that will provide an acceptable exposure indicator number. Suggested techniques are below but may need to be adjusted for the x-ray unit and the digital image receptor being used.
   Exposure #1: 100 mA   150 ms   65 kVp (**Base technique**)
   Exposure #2: **200 mA**   150 ms   65kVp
   Exposure #3: 100 mA   **300 ms**   65 kVp
   Exposure #4: 100 mA   150 ms   **75 kVp**

2. Number each exposure of the knee, and change the technique factors relative to the suggested techniques shown (Be sure to maintain the same collimation throughout):
   a. For Exposure #2, double the mA from the base technique
   b. For Exposure #3, double the time from the base technique
   c. For Exposure #4, increase the kVp by 15% ($\sim$ 10 kVp)

3. Evaluate each image and record the exposure indicator number in the Data Table provided.

4. Repeat Exposures #1 to #4, this time only placing the R-meter in the beam. Record each reading in the Data Table, resetting the meter after each exposure.

5. Analyze the results by answering the questions provided.

Data Table:

Exposure #	Technique		Image Density/Brightness	Exposure Indicator Number	X-Ray Intensity (mR)
	kVp	mAs			
1					
2					
3					
4					

Analysis:

1. **Visually evaluate the radiographic images. Which exposure provided (a) diagnostic image(s)? List them here:**
   A. What change in density (or brightness) was noted in the images with each technique change made? Explain why the image change occurred (or did not occur).

   _____

   _____

   _____

2. Evaluate the exposure indicator numbers for each exposure. Were all of the exposure numbers in the acceptable range for the unit being used? List the exposures that were and were not in the acceptable range.
   A. As each technique change was made, did the exposure number go up or down in value?
   B. Based on your answer to 2A and the direction of the technique change made, is this system's exposure number proportional (in the same direction) as the technique change or inverse (in the opposite direction) of the technique change?

   _____

   _____

   _____

3. Evaluate the x-ray intensity readings for each exposure. What trend(s) do you note with each technique factor change?

   _____

   _____

   _____

4. Compare the exposure indicator number with the mR reading obtained for each exposure. What relationship do you note between these two values for each exposure?
   A. Based on your answer, what relationship can you make between the exposure indicator number and the exposure received by the image receptor?

   _____

   _____

   _____

5. Based on your results, predict what changes would occur in the exposure indicator number and the x-ray intensity values if each technique factor was cut to one-half of the base technique.

   _____

   _____

   _____

6. Using your results, explain how the exposure indicator number can be used to correct an improperly exposed digital image.

   _____

   _____

   _____

Effect of Field Size on X-Ray Beam Intensity, Exposure Values, and Radiation Dose

Name: _____   **Date:** _____

Field size is an important contributor to diagnostic quality and patient dose. Large field sizes create increased scatter radiation by promoting more Compton interactions in patient tissue. Collimation restricts the total number of the patient's atoms interacting with the primary beam, automatically reducing patient dose and scatter. This lab provides students with the opportunity to evaluate the effects of large and small field sizes on beam intensity, exposure indicator values, and image appearance.

Objectives:

Upon the completion of this lab, the student will be able to:

1. Evaluate the effect of field size on radiographic appearance
2. Evaluate the effect of field size on exposure indicator numbers
3. Evaluate the effect of field size on beam intensity
4. Synthesize the relationships between the field size changes and its effects on patient and technologist dose

Materials Needed:

1. Energized radiographic unit
2. Ionization chamber(s) or pocket dosimeter(s)
3. Computed radiographic unit or DR unit
4. Abdomen phantom
5. Lead markers to number each exposure

Procedure:

Exposure #1:

1. Place the abdomen in a lateral position directly on the 14″ × 17″ image receptor on the tabletop (do not use a grid).

2. Center on the lumbar spine and open the collimator to its full 17″ × 17″ size.

3. Expose using the suggested technique (20 mAs at 80 kVp) or another technique provided by your instructor.

4. Process the image, selecting the correct algorithm for a lateral lumbar spine.

5. Using the same technique and field size but without using an image receptor (or deactivating the detector), place a dosimeter on the side of the phantom closest to the collimator, place one dosimeter 1″ behind the spine and a third dosimeter 6″ behind the spine. Take the exposure(s), and record the readings in the Data Table.

Exposure #2:

1. Collimate to a 6″ × 6″ field size, keeping the same centering and technique as Exposure #1.

2. Process the image using the lateral lumbar spine algorithm for the unit.

3. Using the same technique and field size but without using an image receptor (or deactivating the detector), place a dosimeter on the side of the phantom closest to the collimator, place one dosimeter 1″ behind the spine and a third dosimeter 6″ behind the spine. Take the exposure(s), and record the readings in the Data Table.

Data Table:

Acceptable Exposure Indicator Value/Range: _____

Exposure #	Technique		Field Size	Image Brightness	Image Gray Scale	Exposure Indicator Number	X-Ray Intensity (mR) on patient	X-Ray Intensity (mR) 1″ behind	X-Ray Intensity (mR) 6″ behind
	kVp	mAs							
1									
2									

Analysis:

1. Visually inspect the two images. Which image exhibits greater brightness? Longer gray scale?
   A. Explain why the image changes occurred (or did not occur).

   _____

   _____

   _____

2. Evaluate the exposure indicator (EI) values. Which field size indicated an increased exposure to the image receptor?
   A. Explain why the change occurred (or did not occur).

   _____

   _____

   _____

3. Based on your answers to Questions 1 and 2, when critiquing radiographic images, what effect does collimation have on:
   A. Brightness?
   B. Gray scale?
   C. Exposure indicator values?

   _____

   _____

   _____

4. Next, compare the x-ray beam intensity values for each of the exposures. Indicate which exposure had the LOWEST value in each location below:

   On patient: _____

   1″ behind the patient: _____

   6″ behind the patient: _____

   A. Were there any intensity values that did not change or changed relatively little? List them here and explain why the values may not have changed.
   B. Which dosimeter's intensity values changed the most between Exposures #1 and #2?
   C. Calculate the factor of change by dividing the larger intensity value by the smaller intensity value: _____
   D. According to your calculations, by how much (what factor of change) was exposure reduced between the two exposures? _____

   _____

   _____

5. Based on your answers to the questions in #4 above, what effect does collimation have on patient dose? What type of relationship is this?

_____

_____

_____

6. Explain how these results can be used to reduce technologist dose.

_____

_____

_____

Effect of Beam-Part-Image Receptor Alignment on Shape and Size Distortion

Name: _____ **Date:** _____

Fundamental positioning rules require that the central ray be perpendicular to the part and the image receptor and that a minimum of two views 90 degrees to each other should be obtained for each imaging study. However, in some cases, these rules are altered or the x-ray tube is angled due to patient or part position to deliberately change the size or shape of anatomy. This lab will provide students with the opportunity to explore the relationships between the central ray, the anatomic part, and the image receptor, and the effects each change has on elongation, foreshortening, or magnification.

Objectives:

Upon completion of this lab, the student will be able to:

1. Evaluate radiographic images for the presence of shape distortion
2. Evaluate radiographic images for the presence of size distortion
3. Describe how beam-part-image receptor alignment causes either size or shape distortion
4. Synthesize methods to minimize distortion during medical imaging

Materials:

1. Sealed 3″ to 5″ book or box containing flat metal objects*
2. Image receptor
3. Lead numbers

_____

*This needs to be prepared ahead of time by the instructor

Procedure:

1. Determine an appropriate technique (nongrid) or use a technique provided by your instructor. Use this technique for all four exposures.
   Technical Factors: mAs _____ kVp _____ Focal Spot Size: S or L? (circle one)

2. Complete the following four exposures keeping the book or box sealed:
   Exposure #1: Image the object provided using an AP or PA projection.
   Exposure #2: Image the object, standing it on end.
   Exposure #3: Image the object using a 35-degree cephalic angle.
   Exposure #4: Image the object in a dorsal decubitus position.

3. Evaluate the images, identifying which projection each exposure represents, the type of distortion created, and the identity of the objects by completing the table provided. **Do not open or unseal the book or box until you have been instructed to do so.**

4. Open or unseal the box or book and answer the remaining questions.

Data Table:

Exposure #	Appearance, Number, and Size of Objects	Projection or Position (Axial, Tangential, Decubitus, or AP)	Type(s) of Distortion Created	ID of Objects
1				
2				
3				
4				

Analysis:

1. **Evaluate your data and your images. Which projection(s) appeared to cause shape distortion? Which type(s) of distortion was/were created?**
   A. What part of the image geometry was "out of alignment" that created the shape distortion noted?

   _____

   _____

   _____

2. **Which projection(s) appeared to cause size distortion?**
   A. What change in part placement occurred to create this type of distortion?

   _____

   _____

   _____

3. **Were there any projection(s) that appeared to produce radiographs that appeared similar to each other? List them here.**
   A. Explain how the geometry changed and/or did not change to produce these results.
   B. How can this information be used in a clinical setting?

   _____

   _____

   _____

4. **After unsealing the box or book: How accurate were you in identifying all of the objects?**
   A. Which projections helped the most and which projections made it more difficult?
   B. Based on your answers, how can shape distortion be minimized? Size distortion?

   _____

   _____

   _____

Effect of Source-to-Image Receptor Distance (SID) on Magnification and Image Detail

Name: _____   Date: _____

Changes in the source-to-image receptor distance (SID) affect the image receptor exposure, along with geometric properties of the image: specifically spatial resolution (sharpness of detail) and magnification. Generally, the longest SID possible should be used because less penumbra results and magnification is minimized or eliminated. This lab provides students with the opportunity to observe and measure the effects of SID on magnification and detail.

Objectives:

Upon completion of this lab, the student will be able to:

1. Use and interpret a line pair resolution test tool pattern
2. Evaluate radiographic images with different SIDs
3. Analyze the effects of a changed SID on magnification
4. Analyze the effects of a changed SID on spatial resolution (sharpness of detail)

Materials:

1. A small dry bone, such as a phalanx
2. Line pair resolution test pattern (lp/mm)
3. 1″ to 2″ sponge
4. Ruler or tape measure (standard or radiopaque)
5. Image receptor
6. Lead numbers

Procedure:

1. Place the small dry bone and the line resolution test pattern on the sponge on top of the image receptor using a 36″ SID (Exposure #1). Expose using 54 kVp at 0.15 mAs (or another technique that demonstrates adequate density and/or provides an acceptable EI value).

2. For Exposure #2, place the dry bone and line resolution test pattern on the sponge on top of the image receptor using a 72″ SID (Exposure #2). Expose using 54 kVp at 0.6 mAs (or another technique that demonstrates adequate density and/or an acceptable EI value).

3. Using a ruler, measure the length of the bone (in cm) and record where indicated.

4. Analyze the line pair resolution test pattern measurements for each exposure. Record the lp/mm measurement in the Data Table.

5. Using a ruler* and/or the measuring tool available in image processing software, measure the length of the bone (in centimeter) for each exposure. Record each measurement in the Data Table.

6. Calculate the magnification factor of each image by using the formula: MF = imaged bone length/actual bone length. Record in the appropriate column of the Data Table.

7. Analyze the images and answer the questions as indicated.

Data Table:

Original bone length: _____ (cm)

Exposure #	SID (Inches)	Resolution (lp/mm)	Image Bone Length (cm)	Magnification Factor
1				
2				

Analysis:

1. **Visually analyze the edges and the bony trabeculae of each image. Which exposure appears to have the sharpest detail?**

_____

_____

_____

---

*Exposures can also be made using a radiopaque ruler alongside the bone for each image.

2. Compare the lp/mm readings of each exposure. According to your data, which exposure has the highest detail (i.e., highest lp/mm)?

   A. Does this agree with your visual analysis? Why or why not?

   _____

   _____

   _____

3. Compare the bone length measurements and the magnification factor calculations for each exposure. According to your date, which exposure caused the most magnification?

   _____

   _____

   _____

4. Based on your results, complete the following sentence by selecting and inserting the appropriate answer: "To produce radiographs with the highest detail and minimum magnification, a/an _____ (decreased/increased) SID should be used."

   _____

   _____

   _____

Effect of Object-to-Image Receptor Distance (OID) on Magnification and Image Detail

Name: _____   **Date:** _____

The object-to-image receptor distance (OID) plays a major role in size distortion, or magnification, and affects the amount of image blur present in an image. Generally, the shortest OID possible should be used so that less penumbra is produced and magnification is minimized or eliminated. This lab provides students with the opportunity to observe and measure the effects of OID on magnification and spatial resolution (sharpness of detail).

Objectives:

Upon completion of this lab, the student will be able to:

1. Use and interpret a line pair resolution test tool pattern
2. Evaluate radiographic images with different OIDs
3. Analyze the effects of a changed OID on magnification
4. Analyze the effects of a changed OID on image detail

Materials:

1. A small dry bone, such as a phalanx
2. Line pair resolution test pattern (lp/mm)
3. One 1″ sponge and two 3″ to 4″ sponges
4. Ruler or tape measure (standard or radiopaque)
5. Image receptor
6. Lead numbers

Procedure:

1. Place the small dry bone directly on the image receptor and the line resolution test pattern on the 1″ sponge directly beside it. Place on top of the image receptor using a 40″ SID (Exposure #1). Expose using 56 kVp at 0.15 mAs (or another technique that demonstrates adequate density and/or provides an acceptable EI value).

2. Maintain this technique for all three exposures.

3. For Exposure #2, place both the dry bone and line resolution test pattern on the 3″ to 4″ sponge on top of the image receptor. Maintain a 40″ SID.

4. For Exposure #3, place the two 3″ to 4″ sponges on top of each other to create an OID of 6″ to 8″. Place both the dry bone and line resolution test pattern on top of both sponges. Maintain the 40″ SID.

5. Using a ruler* and/or the measuring tool available in image processing software, measure the length of the bone (in centimeter) for each exposure. Record each measurement in the Data Table.

6. Analyze the line pair resolution test pattern measurements for each exposure. Record the lp/mm measurement in the Data Table.

7. Using a ruler, measure the length of the bone (in centimeter) for each exposure. Record each measurement in the Data Table.

8. Calculate the magnification factor of each image by using the formula: MF = imaged bone length/actual bone length. Record in the appropriate column of the Data Table.

9. Analyze the images and answer the questions as indicated.

Data Table:

Original bone length: _____ (cm)

Exposure #	OID (Inches)	Resolution (lp/mm)	Image Bone Length (cm)	Magnification Factor
1				
2				
3				

---

*Exposures can also be made using a radiopaque ruler alongside the bone for each image.

Analysis:

1. Visually analyze the edges and the bony trabeculae of each image. Which exposure appears to have the sharpest detail? The least detail?

_____

_____

_____

2. Compare the lp/mm readings of each exposure. According to your data, which exposure has the highest detail (i.e., highest lp/mm)? The least detail?
   A. Does this agree with your visual analysis? Why or why not?

_____

_____

_____

3. Compare the bone length measurements and the magnification factor calculations for each exposure. According to your date, which exposure caused the most magnification?

_____

_____

_____

4. Based on your results, complete the following sentence by selecting and inserting the appropriate answer: "To produce radiographs with the highest detail and minimum magnification, a/an _____ (decreased/increased) OID should be used."

_____

_____

_____

Effect of Source-to-Image Receptor Distance (SID) on Image Receptor Exposure and Technical Factors

Name: _____   Date: _____

Changes in the source-to-image receptor distance (SID) alter the image receptor exposure and can interfere with the radiographer's ability to obtain a diagnostic image. This is especially true during the performance of mobile radiography. To compensate for SID changes, the direct square law formula has been developed: $mAs_1/mAs_2 = (SID_1)^2/(SID_2)^2$. This lab will examine the effects of distance changes on image receptor exposure and exposure indicator values. It will also provide the student with the opportunity to apply the direct square law when varying distances are used.

Objectives:

Upon completion of this lab, the student will be able to:

1. Convert techniques to compensate for changes in SID
2. Evaluate radiographic images with different SIDs
3. Analyze the effects of a changed SID on image brightness/density
4. Analyze the effects of a changed SID on Exposure Indicator Numbers and x-ray intensity.

Materials:

1. A thorax phantom
2. R-meter, ionization chamber, or pocket dosimeter
3. Tape measure
4. Image receptor
5. Lead numbers

Procedure:

1. Place the thorax phantom at a 72″ (180 cm) SID (Exposure #1), centering for a PA chest exam using a 14″ × 17″ field. Expose using 100 kVp at 5 mAs (or another technique that demonstrates adequate density and/or provides an acceptable EI value).

2. Process this image and all other subsequent images using a PA chest algorithm.

3. For Exposure #2, repeat the exposure using the same technical factors in Exposure #1, but decreasing the SID to 40″ (100 cm).

4. For Exposure #3, use the direct square law to calculate the corrected mAs for 40″ (100 cm). Set the corrected technique and expose the image.

5. Repeat Exposures #1 to #3, this time only placing the ion chamber or dosimeter in the beam. Record each reading in the Data Table, resetting the meter as after each exposure.

6. Note the exposure indicator value of each image, along with its exposure reading in the appropriate column of the Data Table.

7. Analyze the images and answer the questions as indicated.

Data Table:

Acceptable Exposure Indicator Value or Range: _____

Exposure #	Technique		SID (Inches or cm)	Image Density/ Brightness	Exposure Indicator Number	X-Ray Intensity (mR)
	kVp	mAs				
1						
2						
3						

Analysis:

1. Visually evaluate the images produced for Exposures #1 and #2. Which exposure provided (a) diagnostic image(s)? List them here:
   A. What change in density (or brightness) was noted in the images with each technique change made? Explain why the image change occurred (or did not occur).

   _____

   _____

   _____

2. Evaluate the exposure indicator (EI) numbers for Exposures #1 and #2. Were all of the exposure numbers in the acceptable range for the unit being used? List the exposures that were and were not in the acceptable range.

_____

_____

_____

3. Compare the x-ray intensity readings for Exposures #1 and #2. What change in intensity (i.e., image receptor exposure) occurred when SID was changed from 72″ (180 cm) to 40″ (100 cm)?
   A. According to your EI values and intensity readings, was the image receptor under- or overexposed?

_____

_____

_____

4. Compare Exposure #1 with Exposure #3, which used adjusted technique factors to compensate for the SID change. For Image 3, were image density/brightness, the EI value, and the x-ray intensity (i.e., the IR exposure) maintained? In other words, did the direct square law work?
   A. If you answered no, provide a new technique that would work better. (HINT: Use your intensity values to help you determine this.)

_____

_____

_____

5. Evaluate the exposure factors used for Exposures #1 and #3 and their EI and intensity values. What relationship does technique (mAs) have with SID?

_____

_____

_____

Effect of Grids on Exposure Indicator Numbers and Contrast

Name: _____   **Date:** _____

A grid is a radiographic device made of alternating strips of lead and radiolucent materials used to absorb scatter radiation before it reaches the image receptor. The lead strips work to absorb the scatter radiation, while the radiolucent strips allow the more forward traveling photons through to the image receptor. When scatter radiation is absorbed, the exposure to the image receptor is reduced (if no technique compensation is made), but image contrast is increased.

There are various grid ratios available. In order to maintain an adequate number of photons reaching the image receptor when changing from nongrid to a grid exposure, or from grid to grid, the following formula is used:

$$mAs_1 / mAs_2 = GCF_1/GCF_2$$

This lab provides students with the opportunity to observe and measure the effects of nongrid and grid exposures on radiographic exposure and contrast.

Objectives:

Upon completion of this lab, the student will be able to:

1. Convert techniques to compensate for changes in grid ratio
2. Evaluate exposure indicator numbers for adequate IR exposure
3. Visually evaluate radiographs for changes in contrast when different grids are used

Materials:

1. Energized x-ray unit
2. Abdomen or pelvis phantom
3. Two grids of varying grid ratios
4. Image receptors
5. Lead numbers

Procedure:

1. Place the pelvis phantom in an AP position using a bucky or other grid. Place the central ray at the level of the ASIS and centered to the spine. Use a 14″ × 17″ field size or a field size consistent with the grid sizes available. Number the exposure as Exposure #1 and expose the image using the following recommended technique: 80 kVp at 25 mAs (for a 12:1 grid) or a suitable technique to provide adequate brightness and an acceptable exposure indicator number.

2. Convert your Exposure #1 technique using the grid conversion factor formula for the other grid ratio selected. (NOTE: The suggested bucky or grid conversion factors to use for each grid can be found in Table 15.1 of the textbook.)

3. For Exposure #3, use the grid conversion factor formula to determine the technique for a tabletop exposure. Expose and center exactly the same as Exposures #1 and #2.

4. Record the exposure indicator numbers for each image.

5. Analyze the images and answer the questions as indicated.

Data Table:

Expected Exposure Indicator Number or Range: _____

Exposure #	Grid Ratio	mAs	Exposure Indicator #	Image Brightness	Contrast (High or Low)
1					
2					
3					

Analysis:

1. Compare the exposure indicator numbers and the brightness of Exposures #1 and #2. **Were both brightness and exposure indicator number maintained as expected?**
   A. If not, what technique would have worked better? (Use your exposure indicator values to help you determine this.)

   _____

   _____

   _____

2. Compare the exposure indicator numbers and the brightness of Exposures #1 and #3. Were both brightness and exposure indicator number maintained as expected?
   A. If not, what technique would have worked better? (Use your exposure indicator values to help you determine this.)

   _____

   _____

   _____

3. Visually evaluate all of the images. Which image appears to have the highest contrast? The lowest?

   _____

   _____

   _____

4. Explain how adding a grid can improve contrast.

   _____

   _____

   _____

5. What generalization can be made regarding the relationship grid ratios and contrast?

   _____

   _____

   _____

Technique Chart Development

Name: _____   Date: _____

The purpose of standardizing exposure settings is to ensure that diagnostic quality radiographs are obtained every time with minimal radiation exposure to the patient—this includes avoiding repeat exposures. Two fundamental systems for designing technique charts and/or programming anatomically controlled charts are optimum kVp and comparable anatomy. This lab provides an opportunity for students to apply the principles of comparable anatomy and optimal kVp for a preliminary technique chart using actual technique settings and exposures.

Objectives:

Upon completion of this lab, the student will be able to:

1. Perform phantom exposures to acquire a quality image to serve as a reference image and technique for the rest of the chart
2. Apply the 4- to 5-cm rule to alter technique based on patient thickness
3. Use comparable anatomy principles to derive techniques for additional radiographic views and procedures
4. Use the appropriate formulae (i.e., 15% rule or proportional mAs principles) to convert a technique on one anatomical part to another view or procedure.

Materials:

1. Energized x-ray unit
2. 14″ × 17″ image receptor
3. Abdomen phantom
4. Calipers
5. Lead numbers

Procedure:

1. Place the abdomen phantom in an AP position. Measure the patient thickness, and record this measurement in the designated area.

2. Refer to Table 17-2 of the textbook for the optimum kVp setting suggested for an AP abdomen. Set this kVp along with an appropriate mAs to obtain an acceptable exposure indicator number, and a diagnostic image is acquired.
   a. If the initial image is not diagnostic or the EI value is not within range, adjust the technique as needed and repeat the exposure until these requirements are met.

3. Record the information about this exposure in the Data section of this lab.

4. Apply the 4- to 5-cm rule to complete the remainder of the chart for an abdomen examination.

5. To complete the procedure, use comparable anatomy principles to provide technique conversion instructions for another view for this procedure (i.e., an erect abdomen), completing the line provided.

6. Develop techniques for at least two other procedures based on your AP abdomen technique using comparable anatomy principles and answer the Analysis questions.

Data:

Initial Technique Data for an AP abdomen
X-Ray Unit Used: _____   IR System: _____
Procedure: _____   Projection: _____
Technique: SID _____ kVp _____   mAs_____ FSS _____
EI#: _____ Acceptable EI and/or range_____
Grid Ratio _____ (Wall bucky or Table bucky)   Pt. thickness _____ cm
Procedure #1:   __Abdomen__   __AP__ Projection
              _____ kVp   _____ FSS   _____ SID

Thickness							
mAs							

For   __Erect AP__   projection, _____

Procedure #2:   _____   _____ Projection
              _____ kVp   _____ FSS   _____ SID

Thickness							
mAs							

For _____ projection, _____
For _____ projection, _____
For _____ projection, _____

Procedure #3: _____   _____ Projection
                    _____ kVp   _____ FSS   _____ SID

Thickness							
mAs							

For _____ projection, _____
For _____ projection, _____
For _____ projection, _____

Analysis:

1. In an actual department setting, who else should be included in determining the optimum image and starting reference technique?

_____

_____

_____

2. Check the console of the x-ray unit you are using for this technique chart. Are all of the mAs settings listed on your chart available on the machine? If not, what should the technologist do?

_____

_____

_____

3. How could you check the accuracy of your conversions using ALARA principles?

_____

_____

_____

4. When should a technique chart be developed (including programmed anatomically controlled techniques)? When and/or what reasons would indicate that they should be reviewed?

_____

_____

_____

Image Receptors' Effects on Image Blur and Spatial Resolution

Name: _____ Date: _____

The image receptor is responsible for capturing the remnant radiation that exits the patient and converting it to a visible image. The ideal image receptor provides the highest detail possible using the lowest exposure factors. Because the image acquisition process is different for computed radiography (CR) and direct radiography (DR) (and conventional film/screen) systems, their ability to provide spatial resolution, or sharpness of detail, varies also. This lab will investigate the effects of different image receptors on image blur and spatial resolution.

Objectives:

Upon completion of this lab, the student will be able to:

1. Use and evaluate a line pair resolution tool
2. Evaluate radiographs for sharpness of detail and image blur
3. Compare different image receptor systems' effects on spatial resolution and image blur

Materials:

1. Hand phantom
2. Line-pair resolution test tool
3. Computed radiography system and a direct radiography system (and a conventional film/screen system, if available)
4. Energized x-ray unit
5. Lead numbers

Procedure:

1. Position the hand phantom in a PA position directly on a computed radiography image receptor, placing the resolution test pattern beside it **on a 1 inch sponge.**

2. Expose the phantom and resolution test pattern using a technique provided by your instructor to obtain an image of diagnostic quality and an acceptable exposure index number.

3. For Exposure #2, position and expose the hand and resolution test pattern as you did for Exposure #1 using a direct radiography image receptor, using a technique provided by your instructor to obtain an image of diagnostic quality and an acceptable exposure index number.

4. If a conventional film/screen and automatic processing system are available, use this image receptor system for Exposure #3, exposing the hand phantom and resolution test pattern in the same manner as Exposures #1 and #2.

5. Evaluate the images for spatial resolution and image blur.

6. Complete the Data Table and answer the analysis questions as indicated.

Data Table:

IMAGE RECEPTORS AND IMAGE BLUR

Exposure #	Type of Image Receptor System	Image Receptor Speed (If Known)	Resolution (lp/mm)
1			
2			
3			

Analysis:

1. **Visually examine the anatomy and bony trabeculae of the two (or three) exposures. Which exposure appears to have the greatest detail or spatial resolution? The least (i.e., the highest image blur)?**

_____

_____

_____

2. **Refer to the Data Table. Which image receptor resolved the greatest number of line pairs per millimeter? The least?**
   A. Does this agree with your visual observations?

_____

_____

_____

3. Based on your results, which image receptor system provides the greatest sharpness or spatial resolution? The most blur?

_____

_____

_____

4. Describe the difference(s) in each image receptor systems' image acquisition process that would explain why these changes in spatial resolution occur.

_____

_____

_____

Digital Imaging: Exposure Latitude, Exposure Indicator Number QC, and Technique Development

Name: _____   **Date:** _____

Exposure latitude varies from imaging system to imaging system and is what fundamentally controls whether a radiograph is diagnostically acceptable in terms of image quality and/or exposure indicator numbers. Film/screen systems typically had narrower exposure latitudes than digital imaging systems, but this also provided a smaller visual window of acceptable image quality and in turn promoted lower patient dose.

Because digital imaging systems have a wider exposure latitude with quantum mottle providing the only negative effect, increased techniques have been used by technologists to avoid this effect—with no other visible change in image quality—a phenomenon called "dose creep." At the same time, many of the digital systems were/are set up to run as 200 speed imaging systems. Because many departments were using 400 speed film/screen systems prior to their conversion to a digital system, technologists typically converted their techniques by doubling the mAs (which automatically doubled patient dose).

Several experts have proposed decreasing patient dose by increasing kVp using the 15% rule, and cutting the mAs in half, allowing patient dose to be returned to predigital imaging levels or lower. This lab will explore the effect of this type of technique change on digital image quality and x-ray machine output in order to verify that both diagnostic quality and ALARA requirements are met. By evaluating the exposure indicator numbers, image quality, and the exposure latitude of a digital imaging system, students can establish appropriate dose-reducing technique factors.

Objectives:

Upon completion of this lab, the student will be able to:

1. Apply the 15% rule for kVp and the proportional relationship of mAs to convert technical factors
2. Evaluate radiographic images for diagnostic quality

3. Compare the effects of technique changes on image quality, exposure index numbers, and patient exposure/dose
4. Determine the most appropriate technique that provides a diagnostic quality image, an acceptable exposure index number, and the lowest patient dose

Materials:

Abdomen or pelvis phantom

Ionization chamber or R-meter

Computed or Direct radiography system

Procedure:

1. Exposure #1: Expose a pelvis phantom in an AP projection using a digital imaging system using a technique that provides an acceptable exposure index number.
   Suggested technique: _____
   a. Expose the ionization chamber using this technique and record the reading in the appropriate table.

2. Exposure #2: For this exposure, apply the 15% to Exposure #1 so that kVp is increased and adjust the mAs to one-half its original value. (NOTE: Be sure to use the same centering and collimation for each exposure.)
   New technique: _____
   a. Expose the ionization chamber using this technique and record the reading in the appropriate table.

3. Exposure #3: Apply the 15% rule and adjust the technique for Exposure #2 so that kVp is again increased and the mAs is cut in half once more.
   New technique: _____
   a. Expose the ionization chamber using this technique and record the reading in the appropriate table.

4. Exposure #4: Using the digital image receptor, apply the 15% rule again to Exposure #3, with another reduction in mAs.
   New technique: _____
   a. Expose the ionization chamber using this technique and record the reading in the appropriate table.

5. Complete the Data Table as indicated and answer the following analysis questions.

Data Table:

Acceptable Exposure Indicator Number or Range: _____

Exposure #	Technique Used	Exposure Reading (mR)	Exposure Index Number (EIN)
1			
2			
3			
4			

Analysis:

1. Using Image 1 as a baseline, visually compare all of the images. Which of the images appear(s) to have the highest:
   a. Brightness
   b. EIN
   c. Contrast
   d. Noise

   _____

   _____

   _____

2. Are all four images diagnostic? If not, which ones were not, and explain what radiographic quality(ies) is/are no longer optimal.
   A. Were all EIN values in the acceptable range? If not, which ones were not, and explain if they were too high or too low, and if this indicates under- or overexposure.

   _____

   _____

   _____

3. Compare the exposure values for all of the exposures. Which exposure(s) caused the:
   a. Highest exposure
   b. Lowest exposure
   c. Lowest exposure and a diagnostic image

   _____

   _____

   _____

4. Review your answers to Questions 2 and 3. Based on these results, which technique would you recommend be used for an AP pelvis using this x-ray unit and digital imaging system that will provide *both* diagnostic images, an acceptable EIN, and the lowest patient dose?

_____

_____

_____

5. Based on your results and your answers to the analysis questions, are the experts correct? In other words, is using the 15% rule a valid technical tool for reducing patient dose when digital imaging systems are used? Explain why or why not.

_____

_____

_____

Digital Radiography: Image Integrity

Name: _____ **Date:** _____

The advantages that digital imaging systems have over conventional film-screen systems include a wide dynamic range, increased contrast resolution, and the ability to postprocess an image after exposure. However, the workstations and monitors used by the technologist are significantly different than the workstations and monitors used by the radiologist for diagnosis. Generally, the imaging workstations used by the radiologists have a larger matrix, greater contrast resolution capability, and a greater capacity to enhance and manipulate images than the workstations used by the technologists. Due to this, any windowing completed by technologists at their workstations can have a significant effect on the image and its diagnostic value if these changes are saved prior to sending them to the radiologist or diagnosing physician for interpretation.

This lab provides the opportunity for students to observe and compare the images at different workstations and the effects that postprocessing can have on the diagnostic value of the image.

Objectives:

Upon completion of this lab, the student will be able to:

1. Compare the differences in resolution between the workstations and monitors in the general work area with those used by the radiologist for diagnosis
2. Complete basic postprocessing and windowing of a digital image
3. Observe the effects of windowing an image on workstations and monitors in the general work area on the image sent to the high resolution monitor used by the radiologist
4. Describe and compare some of the postprocessing tools and functions available on workstations in the general work area and on the radiologist's high resolution monitor
5. Explain the importance of maintaining the integrity of and sending the original exposed image to the radiologist or interpreting physician without saving postprocessing changes

Materials:

1. Two digital images, preferably on phantoms or images that are not being used for diagnostic purposes
2. General diagnostic monitor and workstation
3. High resolution monitor and workstation

Procedure:

1. Consult with a technologist prior to conducting this lab, ensuring the availability of the radiologist's high resolution monitor and the creation of an artificial patient file for the images being used/created for this laboratory.

2. Follow the instructions and answer the questions.

Data and Analysis:

Before sending a completed radiographic procedure to PACS for diagnosis to the radiologist or interpreting physician, each image must be checked for diagnostic quality.

1. Provide a list of the items checked on each image prior to its being sent electronically for interpretation. Beside each item, describe its parameters and/or guidelines for acceptance.

_____

_____

_____

2. Observe and enhance a digital radiography image at both workstations.
   NOTE: Do NOT save your image enhancements prior to sending it to the radiologist's workstation.
   A. Which workstation appears to have a greater contrast resolution?
   B. Higher detail?
   C. What image enhancement tools are available on the radiologists' workstation that are NOT available on the technologists'?
   D. Utilize some of the image enhancement tools listed. How do the image enhancement tools listed above change the image?
   E. Which workstation images do you feel are more diagnostic? Why?

_____

_____

_____

3. Observe and enhance a digital radiography image at both workstations.
   NOTE: This time, SAVE your image enhancements prior to sending it to the radiologist's workstation.
   A. View the image on the radiologists' workstation. Does it appear different than the first image you sent? Explain.

B. Utilize some of the same image enhancement tools you used above. Describe any changes you notice in the image and/or your ability to manipulate the image compared to your first image.

_____

_____

_____

4. Based on your observations and results, if a digital image has an acceptable exposure indicator number, what image enhancements should a technologist perform and/or save on an image prior to sending it for interpretation?

_____

_____

_____

Digital Imaging Errors or Artifacts

Name: _____   Date: _____

Although there are numerous advantages when digital imaging is used to provide medical images, the appropriate selection and use of technical factors, algorithms, and accessory devices can still affect the quality of the final image. This lab provides students with the opportunity to expose and evaluate radiographic images using both correct and incorrect protocols to determine the effect protocol errors have on image quality and if these errors are able to be corrected using windowing as a postprocessing tool.

Objectives:

Upon completion of this lab, the student will be able to:

1. List some of the causes of radiographic errors or artifacts when digital imaging is used
2. Identify and describe the artifact(s) specific to the imaging problem created during CR/DR use
3. Use and evaluate whether using window or level tools are able to correct the image problem created
4. Describe the corrective action(s) necessary to eliminate the artifact(s) identified

Materials:

Energized x-ray unit

Digital image receptors and workstations

Anatomical phantoms

Procedure:

1. Select one CR or DR problem/incorrect protocol specific to digital imaging from the list below.

2. Using an appropriate phantom and technique, expose the phantom using the correct CR/DR protocol.

3. For your next exposure(s), expose the same phantom using the incorrect protocol you selected.

4. Answer the questions provided.

Digital Imaging Problems/Incorrect Protocols

- Placing more than one exposure field on one imaging plate (CR)

- Placing more than one anatomical part on the detector

- No collimated borders visible on the image receptor

- Using a grid with a frequency in the range of 100 lines/in

- Leaving an imaging plate in the room while other exposures are made

- Exposing an imaging plate or detector upside down

- Collimating down so that < 20% of the image receptor is exposed

- Exposing anatomy with a metal artifact in place (e.g., a surgically implanted pin or nail)

- Displaying four visible collimation borders, but noticeably off-centered on the plate (the anatomy off-centered OR the entire field itself)

- Processing the image using the wrong algorithm (i.e., selecting a chest algorithm for an AP ankle exposure, etc.)

- Other: _____

Protocol Error Selected: _____

Anatomy/Phantom Used: _____   X-Ray Unit Used: _____

Technique Used: _____   Acceptable Exposure Index #: _____

Analysis:

1. **Evaluate the radiographic image exposed under optimum conditions using the appropriate terms:**

   Image Brightness: _____   Contrast: _____

   Noise: _____   Exposure Index #: _____

   Other indicators of image quality (e.g., histogram):

2. **Evaluate the radiographic image exposed using the incorrect image protocol chosen:**

Image Brightness: _____   Contrast: _____

Noise: _____   Exposure Index #: _____

Other indicators:

Describe the artifact(s)/image problem created:

3. **Which indicator(s) in Question 2 above served as the primary cue that the digital image was not adequate? Explain how this indicator was affected.**

4. **Attempt to window and level the image to correct the error. Is the image able to be corrected using these postprocessing tools? Why or why not?**

5. **If the incorrectly exposed image had been taken on an actual patient, explain how it would have to be corrected.**

6. **Which computed radiography image/equipment/software function(s) and/or components were "misled" by the erroneous exposure conditions?**

7. **How can the artifact(s)/image problem you created be prevented from occurring?**

8. **Based on your lab results and experience, which of the following imaging and positioning factors are still the responsibility of the technologist when digital imaging systems are used? (Check all that apply.)**

_____ kVp selection   _____ mAs Selection

_____ Photocell selection   _____ Grid Use

_____ Anatomic part selection _____ SID Selection

_____ Appropriate centering   _____ Correct Positioning

_____ R and L Markers   _____ Patient Identification

_____ Collimation   _____ Patient Instructions

Fluoroscopy and C-arms: Components of Image Intensified Fluoroscopy Systems

Name: _____   **Date:** _____

Fluoroscopy is a dynamic imaging modality designed to observe moving structures in the body, in contrast to conventional radiography that produces static images of body structures. This imaging method allows the radiologist or other physicians to observe physiological functions and the proper placement of medical devices during surgical procedures. The technologist is often called to assist and/or operate the fluoroscope, so it is important that s/he be knowledgeable of the controls and functions of this device.

Objectives:

Upon completion of this lab, the student will be able to:

1. Identify the controls of a stationary fluoroscope and describe their functions
2. Identify the controls of a mobile fluoroscope and describe their functions
3. Compare and contrast the controls and functions of a stationary and mobile fluoroscope
4. Describe the imaging chain, listing all of the energy conversions which occur prior to obtaining a visible image

Materials:

1. A stationary fluoroscopic unit (and operator's manual, if needed)
2. A mobile fluoroscopic unit (and operator's manual, if needed)

Procedure:

1. Follow the instructions and answer the questions provided.

Data and Analysis:

Part A:

Below is a diagram of a patient on a radiographic examination table. Draw and label the following components:

1. X-ray tube
2. Image Intensifier
3. Carriage or "C-arm"
4. Video camera tube or CCD
5. Monitor

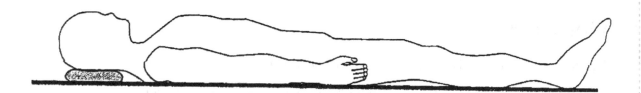

Answer the following questions based on your drawing and the information covered in the textbook:

1. **Where is the source of radiation located in reference to the patient?**

   _____

   _____

   _____

2. **If a gonad shield was used, where should it be placed to protect the patient?**

   _____

   _____

   _____

3. Where is the "image receptor" in this case?

_____

_____

_____

4. Trace the imaging chain from the x-ray tube (primary radiation) to the monitor (visible light) by listing the components traveled through and the conversions made from one form of energy to another.

_____

_____

_____

Part B:

1. Diagram and label the operator's panel of a stationary fluoroscopy unit below.

2. Underneath your diagram, briefly describe the function of each button or switch.

_____

_____

_____

Part C:

1. Diagram and label the operator's panel of a mobile fluoroscopy unit (C-arm) below.

2. Underneath your diagram, briefly describe the function of each button or switch.

_____

_____

_____

3. List the similarities of the two units' controls and functions, along with any differences where indicated below:

Similarities	Differences
_____	_____
_____	_____
_____	_____

Fluoroscopy and C-arm Use: Fluoroscopic Image Quality and the Automatic Brightness Control System

Name: _____   Date: _____

Fluoroscopy is a dynamic imaging modality that allows live moving structures to be imaged and observed. Although this imaging method allows the direct observation of physiological functions, radiographic image quality is sacrificed. Because the fluoroscope is often moved during a procedure, the unit must be able to compensate for changes in body thickness so that each body structure can be visualized during the examination. The device that allows this to occur is called the Automatic Brightness Control System.

This lab will provide students with the opportunity to operate a stationary and/or mobile fluoroscopic system, evaluate the quality of the images produced, and observe the operation of the Automatic Brightness Control System during fluoroscopy.

Objectives:

Upon completion of this lab, the student will be able to:

1. Safely operate a stationary or mobile fluoroscope
2. Determine the technical factors typically used during fluoroscopy
3. Evaluate the radiographic quality of fluoroscopic images
4. Describe the effects of Automatic Brightness Control on the image during fluoroscopy

Materials:

1. A stationary or mobile fluoroscopic unit (and operator's manual, if needed)
2. A radiographic examination table
3. Hip, shoulder, thorax, or abdominal phantom
4. Lead aprons

Procedure:

1. Have everyone who will be participating in the lab put on a lead apron.

2. Perform the necessary start-up procedures for the fluoroscopy unit.

3. Under supervision, operate the fluoroscope as described and answer the questions provided.

Data and Analysis:

Place the phantom underneath the image intensifier of a stationary or mobile fluoroscopy unit. Have one person operating the fluoro, and another at the control panel to note the conditions of the exposure. Depress the exposure switch briefly, while noting the following:

1. **List the technical factors (kVp/mA/time) and their settings that are displayed while fluoro is engaged:**
   A. How do the technical factors you listed above compare to conventional overhead techniques?

   _____

   _____

   _____

2. **While fluoroscopy is in progress, what indicator(s) is/are present that fluoro is "on"?**

   _____

   _____

   _____

   Begin fluoro again. While watching the monitor, open and close the collimators.

3. **Describe what changes occurred in the image in terms of density (brightness), contrast, and noise/fog when the collimators were changed.**

   _____

   _____

   _____

4. Overall, in terms of sharpness of detail, how does the image on the monitor compare with the same image if it were a static radiographic image?

_____

_____

_____

5. View the image on the monitor again, both from a normal viewing distance and up close to the screen. You should note that the image appears grainy. What is the radiographic term for this quality? What causes it to occur?

_____

_____

_____

Resume fluoro again, moving the carriage so that the phantom is centered to the image. Move the carriage and/or table slowly from the center of the phantom to one side, observing the image closely during the motion. Return the carriage slowly to the center of the phantom and then move it (or the table) gradually up or down until the phantom disappears from the image.

6. Describe how the image changes as the fluoroscope moves from a thick portion of the phantom to a thin region.

_____

_____

_____

7. Identify the mechanism that causes the changes in Question 6, and briefly describe how it works.

_____

_____

_____

Collimator Quality Control: Field Size and Light Field Alignment

Name: _____   **Date:** _____

Collimator quality control testing is an important component of medical imaging QC that a technologist can perform on a periodic basis and/or whenever a problem with the light field is suspected. If the collimator light is out of alignment from the x-ray field, the technologist risks clipping anatomy, and this leads to repeat exposures. Because of the configuration of the light and the mirrors used in collimators, abrupt changes in the orientation of the tube head from vertical to horizontal can cause the alignment of the light field to no longer be congruent with the x-ray field. Due to this, this quality control test should be performed on a biannual basis.

Objectives:

Upon completion of this lab, the student will be able to:

1. Describe and use the equipment needed to conduct field size quality control testing.
2. List and describe acceptance and quality control parameters for collimation and field size.
3. Measure and evaluate radiographic images for compliance with field size quality control requirements.
4. Explain why field size quality control testing should be performed.

Materials:

1. Lead or radiopaque ruler(s) (e.g., Supertech)
2. Standard ruler or tape measure
3. Energized x-ray unit
4. Image receptor (10″ × 12″ if using a CR imaging plate)
5. Calculator

Procedure:

1. With the SID at 40″ (100 cm), place a 10″ × 12″ CR imaging plate directly on the x-ray table top, or if testing a DR system, proceed directly to Step 2.

2. Collimate well within the edges of the CR cassette or to a nominal 8″ × 10″ field size for a DR system.

3. Measure the light field and note the collimator settings and insert this information where indicated in Question 1 of the Analysis section.

4. Open the (SuperTech) rulers so that each ruler is 90 degrees to each other (or lay two radiopaque rulers 90 degrees to each other). Align the center screw of the rulers (or the midpoint of the two individual rulers) with the central ray of the light field. Use lead letters to designate each side of the image as N, S, E, W.

5. Place two coins* on each side of the light field (a total of eight coins), with the edge of each coin intersecting at the light field edge.

6. Expose using an extremity tabletop technique and process the image using an extremity algorithm.

7. Evaluate each edge of the image and answer the analysis questions, using your data.

   *Nickels are 2 cm in diameter, and this, along with the rulers, can be used to quickly estimate any misalignment based on the nickel on the inside or outside of the x-ray beam.

Analysis:

1. **Note the collimator setting and measure the actual size of the light field on the image receptor.**
   a. Collimator setting: Length = _____(in or cm), width = _____ (in or cm)
   b. Light field: Length = _____(in or cm), width = _____ (in or cm)

2. **Measure the actual x-ray field using the exposed rulers on a monitor and record below:**
   a. X-ray field: Length = _____ (in or cm), width = _____ (in or cm)

3. **What is the acceptable limit for field size accuracy?**

   _____

   _____

   _____

4. Are these within the limits of acceptability?

_____

_____

_____

5. For each edge of the x-ray field, measure how far the edge of the black exposed area is from the light field markers and in which direction. List your results below:
   a. North side = _____ cm off to _____ (direction)
   b. South side = _____ cm off to _____ (direction)
   c. East side = _____ cm off to _____ (direction)
   d. West side = _____ cm off to _____ (direction)

6. Divide each of the deviation measurements in number 5 above by the SID (100 cm) and multiply this result by 100 to obtain the percentage deviation from the SID and record below:
   a. North side = _____ % of SID off
   b. South side = _____ % of SID off
   c. East side = _____ % of SID off
   d. West side = _____ % of SID off

7. What is the limit of acceptable deviation for light field edge alignment with the actual x-ray field?

_____

_____

_____

8. Which, if any, of the light field edges are out of alignment by unacceptable amounts?

_____

_____

_____

9. For any measurement that was not in compliance, what negative effects would result if this problem is not corrected?

_____

_____

_____

Digital Radiography Quality Control Activity Log

Name: _____   **Date:** _____

A digital imaging department's components require regular quality control monitoring to ensure diagnostic quality images. These include: (1) the laser reader; (2) the image display workstation, (3) the computed radiography (CR) and digital radiography (DR) imaging equipment/imaging plates; and (4) the picture archiving communication system. This lab provides the student with the opportunity to observe and participate in the quality control of the department.

Objectives:

Upon completion of this lab, the student will be able to:

1. List the various QC actions taken on a daily, monthly, or other systematic basis in a digital imaging environment
2. Explain the importance of conducting regular QC testing of digital imaging equipment
3. Describe the QC actions taken regarding the care and maintenance of imaging plates, a DR system, the PACS network, and the image display workstation
4. Observe and participate in available CR/DR QC activities

Procedure:

During a period of one month or other monitoring period as designated by your instructor, you will be:

1. Investigating what regular QC tests are conducted in a digital imaging department and/or discovering what additional tests may be completed. Document your results by completing the table and answering the questions in Part I of this lab.

2. Documenting the results of your participation in various QC activities. Complete the table in Part II of this lab and answer the questions.

Data and Analysis:

Part I: Digital Imaging QC Activities

1. What activities are conducted by the department to ensure the accurate acquisition and display of images on the imaging plates and the imaging workstations? Complete the table below as indicated.

   NOTE: You may have already observed some of these activities; others you may need to obtain by interviewing the department's designated PACS/QC personnel.

CR Component: QC Action or Test	Accuracy Requirements	Frequency	Who Conducts/ Other Information
CR PLATES AND/OR DR PANEL			
1.			
2.			
VIDEO MONITOR/ WORKSTATION			
1.			
2.			
LASER READER, PRINTER, AND/ OR PACS SYSTEM			
1.			
2.			

2. After completing the table, select ONE item from EACH category and explain how the completion of this test or activity ensures an optimum image and/or maintains the optimal operation of the system/department (i.e., What would happen if this activity was NOT completed?)

   _____

   _____

   _____

   _____

   _____

   _____

Data and Analysis:

Part II: QC Activity Log

1. During the QC period, you will need to document your participation in and/or observation of various CR/DR/PACS QC activities. It is desirable that you participate in as many of these activities as possible. However, a one-time demonstration of some of the activities conducted on a less frequent basis is also acceptable. Log your activities on the attached table to be turned in at the end of the period.

Log of Quality Control Activities

During the QC period, document your observation of and/or participation in the department's QC activities using the table below.

Date	Activity	Observed or Participated	Date	Activity	Observed or Participated

Summary

1. Which activities did you engage in the most?

_____

_____

_____

_____

2. List any problems you encountered and/or potential problems you were able to prevent due to your activities.

_____

_____

_____

_____

_____

3. Briefly describe your impressions of the state of QC in radiology with regard to DR, CR, and PACS as a result of this lab activity.

_____

_____

_____

_____

_____

Repeat/Reject Analysis

Name: _____   Date: _____

An important component of a quality control program is monitoring repeat exposures and reject images. By identifying trends in repeat/reject exposures, a department can determine the causes of the repeat or reject exposures and take steps to correct the identified problems. By eliminating repeat exposures, a department can save time and money and reduce patient exposure. This lab provides students with the opportunity to track and analyze their own repeat or reject exposures.

Objectives:

Upon completion of this lab, the student will be able to:

1. Calculate his/her repeat rate for the entire period
2. Calculate his/her repeat rate by cause
3. Calculate his/her repeat rate by exam category
4. Identify trends and possible causes of his/her repeat exposures
5. Synthesize strategies and solutions to improve his/her repeat rate

Materials:

1. Daily Procedure Record (additional copies may need to be made to cover the full reporting period)
2. Repeat Analysis Worksheet
3. Calculator

Procedure:

1. For a period of 1 month, or as directed by your instructor, record all of your repeat radiographs regardless of cause.

2. During this time period, keep accurate records of the total number of views taken, completing Chart A (Daily Procedure Record) for every procedure. (Note: You are to record the number of **exposures or views** taken, **not** simply the number of films/imaging plates used.)

3. At the end of the data collection period, complete Chart B (Repeat Analysis Worksheet) by transferring the total number of exposures (views) taken each day into appropriate categories. Add the totals together as directed to determine the grand totals for the period in each period.

4. Answer the questions as indicated.

Results and Analysis:

1. Total your Daily Procedure Record. Record the grand total number of views taken:_____

2. Record the total number of repeat exposures made here: _____

3. To calculate your overall repeat rate, divide the total number of repeat exposures taken for the period by the grand total number of views. Multiply the result by 100.

   Overall repeat rate: _____%

4. Next, examine and tally the primary causes of your repeats and sort into each of the categories below. Record the number of repeats in each group:

Reason for Repeat	**Number of Repeats**
Positioning	_____
Overexposed	_____
Underexposed	_____
Motion	_____
Artifacts on patient, film, or table/processing	_____
Other: Collimation or alignment (centering)	_____
TOTAL:	_____

5. Compute your causal repeat rate as follows: Divide the number of repeats for each reason by **the total number of repeats** for the period. Multiply the result by 100. Record your repeat rate for each category below:

Positioning	_____%
Overexposed	_____%
Underexposed	_____%
Motion	_____%
Artifacts on patient, film, or table/processing	_____%
Other: Collimation or alignment (centering)	_____%

6. Which type of problem caused the most repeat exposures? The second-most?

7. If you were a supervisor, what actions would you initiate in your department to reduce the type of repeats listed above if this was a department-wide problem? (Think of at least two different strategies to ensure improvement.)

8. Next, look over your Repeat Analysis Worksheet to evaluate your repeats by exam category. To calculate your repeat rate, divide the number of repeats taken for each procedure by the total number of repeats for the period. Multiply each result by 100% and record in the % column on the far right of the Worksheet.

9. Which exams/procedures had the highest repeat rate? Second-highest?

10. If you were a supervisor, what actions would you initiate in your department to reduce the type of repeats listed above if this was a department-wide problem? (Think of at least two different strategies to ensure improvement.)

Chart A: Daily Procedure Record

For each date of data collection, complete each column calculating the number of views expected and actually taken.

Date	Exam	Routine # of Views Taken	Actual # of Views Taken	# or Views Repeated/Cause
	Total for this date:			

Date	Exam	Routine # of Views Taken	Actual # of Views Taken	# or Views Repeated/Cause
	Total for this date:			

Chart B: Repeat Analysis Worksheet

Using the Daily Procedure Record, complete the chart below by tranferring the total number of **repeat exposures (views).**

SURVEY PERIOD: _____ TO _____ LOCATION(S): _____

Category Exam	Position	Overex-posed	Underex-posed	Motion	Artifacts	Other	Total	%
Chest								
Ribs								
Shoulder								
Humerus								
Elbow								
Forearm								
Wrist								
Hand								
C-Spine								
T-Spine								
L-spine								
Skull								
Facial								
Sinuses								
Abdomen								
Pelvis								
Hip								
Femur								
Knee								
Tib/Fib								
Ankle								
Foot								
UGI								
Esophagram								
SBFT								
BE								
IVU								
Other								
TOTAL								
TOTAL %								

Protective Apparel Quality Control

Name: _____   **Date:** _____

As part of a total quality assurance program in a medical imaging department, all of the protective apparel should be checked to ensure the lead aprons, gloves, and thyroid shields are intact and safe to use. This quality control check should be performed annually and includes both a visual and radiographic inspection. This lab provides the student with the opportunity to perform this quality control test.

Objectives:

Upon completion of this lab, the student will be able to:

1. Describe the frequency and parameters of acceptance for protective apparel quality control
2. Perform a visual inspection of protective apparel to identify any defects and describe the required actions taken if any defects are found
3. Perform a radiographic inspection of protective apparel (either using fluoroscopy or by taking radiographic images) to identify any defects and describe the required actions taken if any defects are found
4. Complete the required documentation for this quality control test.

Materials:

1. Energized x-ray or fluoroscopic unit
2. Lead aprons and other protective apparel, lettered or numbered for tracking and documentation purposes

Procedure:

1. Inspect the lead aprons or other protective apparel physically for any obvious damage like tears, seams that are unraveling, perforations, or thinning creases. Record your results in the Data Table.

2. Examine the aprons and other apparel that passed the physical test radiographically. If fluoroscopy is used, set the unit to a manual technique setting. Do not use the automatic brightness control because this will produce additional unwanted radiation.

3. Evaluate the fluoroscopic or radiographic images to determine if there is damage such as rotting or vampire marks (tiny holes resembling teeth marks). Under fluoroscopy, the shielded areas will be dark, and the defects, seams, and stitching will appear light on the images. The reverse will be true if radiographing the aprons and other apparel. Record your results in the Data Table and answer the Analysis questions.

4. NOTE: If using fluoroscopy, once you have "cleared" a lead apron under fluoroscopy, wear that apron and fluoro the next apron(s).

Data Table:

LEAD PROTECTIVE APPAREL SURVEY

Date of Survey: _____

Apron Inventory Number	Color	Visual Inspection Results	Fluoroscopy Inspection Results	Pass/Fail	Comments

Analysis:

1. Evaluate your data. Did all of the aprons pass the inspection? List those aprons that passed and those that did not.

_____

_____

_____

2. If a lead apron or other protective device does not pass inspection, what actions must a technologist and medical imaging department take?

_____

_____

_____

3. What are the regulatory requirements to safely dispose of a lead apron or other accessory device if it is found to be defective?

_____

_____

_____

4. How often should this quality control check be conducted?

_____

_____

_____